Best Little Beginner Fat Burning Book
Easiest Fastest Tips to Burn Fat
By Chris Joseph
Copyright 2015
If you enjoyed learning the information in this book... you may also be interested in...
These other titles by Chris Joseph
9 Day Smoothie Cleansing Diet
If you have been helped by purchasing this book please take a minute by letting me know how it helped you by leaving a review at the bookseller where you purchased your book.
I am always interested to know how my readers are doing and what successes they are having.
Wishing you a healthy day!
Chris Joseph

Laws of Fat-Burning

Our bodies are fat-burning machines. It all comes down to metabolism: the chemical process involved in processing nutrients, eliminating wastes, and producing the energy necessary for growth and life. Plants convert the energy of the sun into glucose which our bodies then proceed to break down back into usable energy. Some of the food we eat is immediately burned for energy and some is stored as fat for future energy use.

We are constantly burning calories and fat for our daily energy needs but the rate at which we burn through calories differs based on genetics, hormonal activity, digestion and exercise. Thus, you must consume fewer calories than you burn and keep your metabolism active and hormone levels even through appropriate exercise, healthy eating and sleep. In general, you must avoid simple sugars and processed foods. And, most importantly, in order to prevent increased fat retention, you must lose weight gradually.

Lose weight gradually

Considering your metabolism, it is important to lose weight gradually. You should neither drastically cut your calorie consumption nor lose too much weight at once. When you skip a meal or diet, actually if you go more than 4-5 hours without eating, your blood sugar becomes unstable. So, when you do eat, your insulin levels will spike and, regardless of what you eat, your body stores it as fat.

After much research, we have learned that a 10% decrease in body weight will result in a reduced metabolism that effectively aims to gain back the fat lost if not more. After weight loss, the individual is metabolically different from a person naturally at the same weight and activity level.

Muscle fibers also adapt to perform more efficiently, burning 20-25% fewer calories during exercise. Basically, after dieting, in order to maintain the new weight, people must eat 250-400 calories less than their counterparts who had not dieted and burn fewer calories in the same activity (i.e. 150 calories instead of 200 calories when walking). Likewise, the brain induces cravings and suppresses resistance to high-calorie foods. The body will actually continue to defend the higher weight for as many as six years. So, as hard as it is to accept, gradual weight loss is the first law of fat burning.

Keep your metabolism active

Metabolism can be divided into three types: basal or resting metabolism, digestive metabolism and exercise or movement metabolism. Resting and digestive metabolism uses the majority of the calories burned every day. The amount of energy used in eating also varies based on what is being eaten. It takes more energy to digest protein and fiber than it does carbohydrates and fat. Also, eating more not less will elevate and quicken your metabolism.

Get your metabolism started off right with a good breakfast and then eating a healthy snack or small meal every three hours. You can continue eating exactly the same amount split up over more meals and naturally store less of it as fat and burn more of it for energy without extra work (Marteski).

Avoid simple carbohydrates, processed foods and beverages with added sugar, as well as fat-free products that compensate for flavor with sugar. Without fat, sugar is absorbed into the blood even faster (Bass). Protein and fiber also slows digestion and gradually increases, instead of spikes, blood sugar levels. Omega 3 fatty acids will also help maintain stable insulin levels.

This is the most effective way to keep your metabolism high, prevent hunger pangs and binges. Simple sugars and processed foods also have other consequences on the balance of hormones that affect metabolism and fat loss.

Moreover, the body's resting metabolism is negatively affected by a larger ratio of fat to muscle in the body. Muscle is more metabolically active than fat. It burns three times as many calories as fat to sustain itself, primarily drawing on energy stores in fat (Women's Health).

Not all fat is made equal nor is it as easy to spot as you would think. Visceral fat, which cushions the organs inside your abdominal cavity, is less apparent and much more involved in producing hormones that affect metabolism, fat storage, and hunger.

There is a correlation between more visceral fat and less adiponection, a hormone that regulates metabolism, thus lowering metabolism. While exercise can only target 15-30% of your daily calorie burn, strength building exercises will burn fat in order to build muscle—muscle which will increase your basal metabolism as well.

It is also important to vary the kinds of exercise, how long and how hard your workout, particularly when it comes to cardio. The body quickly adapts to cardiovascular exercise, so you will find yourself spending more time running on the treadmill with diminishing returns. In order to prevent this kind of stagnation, change up how long you exercise, when you exercise and the types of exercise.

Try out the treadmill one day and the rowing machine the next. Go for a run every morning and then scale down the daily jogs the next week. Mix in full body workouts that build strength and muscle. Work interval training into your exercise time. This will keep your workouts effectively burning muscle and not just effectively using calories to perform the same daily routine activity.

Build muscle

As mentioned before, muscle burns fat and increases your metabolism. In fact, muscle is catabolic meaning that it burns calories even when it's not active. Unfortunately, as we age, we lose a fifth of a pound of muscle a year, even more after age 50 (Marteski).

Combined with a slowing metabolism, loss of muscle negatively affects the immune system, the body's ability to respond to stress, as well as the strength of bones and joints. Protein and exercise that incorporates strength and interval training are essential to building and maintaining muscle strength. Protein not only is necessary for building muscle but it also slows sugar absorption and your rate of digestion which is good for your metabolism.

The ideal ratio of protein, carbohydrate and fat is 40:40:20. However, remember to choose the best sources of these nutrients. Beans, often overlooked in favor of meat, eggs and dairy, are rich in protein as well as fiber. Also, whole grains and monounsaturated fats are preferred over simple sugars and saturated and Trans fats.

Keep your hormones balanced: cortisol, leptin, ghrelin, and insulin

Fat cells, especially abdominal fat cells, are biologically active producing "lots of nasty substances" including fat hormones, hunger hormones and stress hormones (Collins). IN particular, fat cells produce leptin that suppresses appetite and regulates ghrelin, another hormone that signals hunger and cravings to the brain (Magee).

Chronic stress and sleep deprivation also increase the levels of these hormones. Besides this, your blood sugar level affects how energetic or hungry you feel. It also tells your body whether to burn fat or store it. When your blood sugar level increases, your pancreas produces insulin to help regulate the sugar in your blood. Higher levels of insulin tell your body that you have plenty of energy and to store fat instead of burning it.

Since insulin is the fat storage hormone, it is actually impossible to burn body fat with the surge of insulin that comes from consuming sugar. The resulting sugar crash will leave you feeling tired and hungry, and our bodies respond by craving more sugar.

Over time, the body becomes less sensitive to leptin and insulin, producing extra insulin, and using sugar more often for fat storage instead of energy. The body also produces less adiponectin as belly fat increase. Fat cells also produce the stress hormones, cortisol, and inflammatory substances, like cytokines, that regulate metabolism and the immune system.

Losing fat is a combination of calorie intake, types of calories, metabolism, calorie burning and timing. If a person eats fewer calories than needed daily, the body will get its energy by burning through its fat storage. However, the body will also adapt by slowing its metabolism, reducing how much energy it needs to survive, and altering its hormonal balance.

Even a 10% decrease in body weight will result in a metabolically different person compared to a person naturally at the same weight and activity level. Muscle fibers also change making them more efficient and thus burning 20-25% fewer calories during exercise. At the same time, the brain induces cravings and suppresses resistance to high-calorie foods.

In order to outwit your body, you must keep the basic laws of fat-burning in mind as you approach fat loss. You cannot drastically cut your calories or cut out carbohydrates all together because your body will not only stop burning fat but it will store it instead.

In order to burn fat, you have to think of how eating, exercising and even sleeping affects your metabolism. An active, balanced and healthy metabolism burns fat for you for optimum fitness and health. If you treat your body right, it will do everything it can to be strong and healthy.

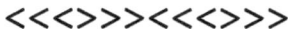

The truth about fat loss

Regardless of the diet plan, the weight returns. However, there are 10,000 people on the National Weight Control Registry that have succeeded at keeping the weight off. People on the registry have all lost 30 pounds or more, on average 70, and kept it off for at least a year, on average six years!

Common to all these people is their hyper vigilance: to keep off the weight, they must exercise more and eat less than someone who maintains that weight naturally. They eat less, 50-300 fewer daily calories, more consistently, never breaking their food choice and eating patterns.

They weigh themselves every day. They watch less television, as little as half, and exercise more, an hour or more a day and walking on average the equivalent of four miles every day. In order to maintain their lower rate, they cannot let up for years!

Tara Parker-Pope, health writer for The Times, describes several success stories in her cover story "The Fat Trap," one of who is Janice Bridge. After years of dieting starting at age 14, she reduced her weight from 330 pounds to 195 pounds, with a low of 165 pounds, over three years, with the help of a medically supervised weight loss program and an 800 calorie diet. It is only through her hyper vigilance that she has been able to maintain this 135-pound weight loss for five years.

She weighs all food, calculates the exact number of calorie, and reviews online menus to calculate calories before going out to eat. She avoids food that prompts her cravings and overeating, and she keeps a food journal to account for her total calories and protein every day. She also drinks 100 ounces of water and exercises for 2 hours every day.

Using years of exercise and diet data, she has calculated how many calories her body personally burns. While the average person uses 11 calories per minute when biking, Janice burns 4-5 calories a minute while biking. In order to maintain her weight, she can eat 2,000 calories and burn 500 calories in exercise. To account for errors, she allows herself 1,800 calories while a similarly active woman of her age and size can eat about 2,300 calories. This is not unusual for people who have managed to maintain their weight loss (Parker-Pope, 2011).

To understand the truth about fat loss, we need to clarify what fat is

Fat, or adipose tissue, is necessary to cushion the body's internal organs. Body fat is the percentage of a person's body that is fat and not water, muscle, bone or vital organs. The normal healthy young men have 15% body fat and for women 27%, increasing by 5% in adulthood. Of that 3% for men is essential fat in tissues and organs including bone marrow, the nervous system and muscle. For women, due to reproductive needs, this percentage is higher: 12%.

Fat is vital to normal structure and function (Segen's Medical Dictionary, 2012). It is also an energy reserve for the body (Dorland's Medical Dictionary, 2007). Storage fat is the energy reserve that "accumulates as adipose tissue beneath the skin and in visceral depots." This is 12% body mass for men and 15% body mass for women (Medical Dictionary for the Health Professions and Nursing, 2012).

Research has found a genetic predisposition for or against obesity. The findings of Canadian researchers Claude Bouchard and Angelo Tremblay suggest that "biological determinism" can make a person susceptible to weight gain or loss.

They studied 31 pairs of male twins, aged 17-29, with no family history of obesity. Twins were fed 84,000 calories beyond their basic needs over 120 days which should have resulted in a 24 pound weight gain. However, while weight gain and fat distribution was similar between twins, some twins gained less than 10 pounds while others gained 30 with three times as much belly fat.

This genetic disposition was also apparent in exercise studies involving weight loss. As of October 2010, 32 distinct genetic variations associated with obesity or body-mass index have been confirmed. People who carry a variant known as FTO face a 30% higher risk of obesity and 60% higher if they have two FTO variants. The FTO variant is more common among people with a European or African background (65%) compared to those of an Asian background (27-44%). Studies also suggest the trait influences eating habits (Bouchard & Tremblay, 1990).

In order to lose weight, you must use more calories than consumed daily

The U.S. Department of Agriculture and U.S. Department of Health and Human Services stated: "Calorie balance over time is the key to weight management. Calorie balance refers to the relationship between calories consumed from foods and beverages and calories expended in normal body functions (i.e., metabolic processes) and through physical activity. People cannot control the calories expended in metabolic processes, but they can control what they eat and drink, as well as how many calories they use in physical activity" (Dietary Guidelines for Americans, 2010).

Building cells, moving muscles, and maintaining body temperature all requires energy. How many calories you need daily depends on weight, age, activity and metabolic rate. Metabolism is all of the chemical processes involved in the bodily functions of growth, waste elimination, and distribution of nutrients. The metabolic rate can be affected by exercise, body temperature, hormonal activity and digestion.

In general, the body uses only the amount of energy from its daily intake that it needs for energy purposes and stores the remainder as fat (Mosby's Medical Dictionary, 2003). So, if a person eats more calories than needed daily the person will gain weight. If he or she eats fewer calories than needed daily, "the body will supplement its energy sources by drawing upon stores of fat" and he or she will lose weight (Quoted in Parker-Pope, 2011).

Dieting can negatively affect your metabolism

The reason most people gain back the weight they have lost has absolutely nothing to do with willpower. Joseph Proietto, a physician at the University of Melbourne, studied 50 obese men and women who lost an average of 30 pounds over ten weeks with a 500-550 calorie diet.

Though patients received nutritional counseling and encouragement to exercise and eat healthily, patients regained an average of 11 pounds within a year. They also were more hungry and preoccupied with food than before the weight loss.

This is due to the metabolic and hormonal changes that result from weight loss. The bodies of these men and women remained in a biologically altered state working overtime to regain the lost weight.

Even though they were no longer on a 500 calorie diet their bodies continued to act like they were starving. Hormones associated with hunger were higher, suppressing hunger lower, and increasing metabolism also lower compared to before the original diet.

Due to the weight loss, these people suffer from a unique metabolic state post-diet wherein the body was fighting to gain back the lost weight (Proietto, 2011). Other research shows that a 10% decrease in body weight will result in a metabolically different person compared to a person naturally at the same weight and activity level.

Muscle fibers also change making them more efficient and thus burning 20-25% fewer calories during exercise. Basically, after dieting, in order to maintain the new weight, the person has to consume 250-400 calories less than their counterparts who have not dieted and he or she will be burning 150 calories walking instead of 200 calories. Likewise, the brain induces cravings and suppresses resistance to high-calorie foods.

"After you've lost weight, your brain has a greater emotional response to food," Rosenbaum says. "You want it more, but the areas of the brain involved in restraint are less active...you've created the perfect storm for weight regain" (Quoted in Parker-Pope, 2011). The body will continue to defend the higher weight for as many as six years.

The truth about fat loss is that without gradual weight loss and hyper vigilance the fat is likely to come back. There is a period of time wherein a person can gain and lose weight without altering their current metabolism.

This depends on genetic risk for obesity and the amount of time the person carried the extra weight before trying to lose it. Despite temporary weight gain during the holidays, college, and even actors in different roles, we see that people clearly can put the weight back on or shed the pounds without altering their daily caloric needs.

In mice, the window is eight months. Rudolph Leibel, an obesity researcher at Columbia University in New York, says "Before that time, a fat mouse can come back to being a skinny mouse again without too much adjustment. For a human we don't know, but I'm pretty sure it's not measured in months, but in years." In general, without further scientific gains, gradual weight lost is by far more sustainable than fast weight loss.

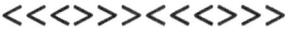

Top fat loss mistakes people make

The most common fat loss mistakes involve a misunderstanding of fat, dieting, exercise, sugar and food. The body's fat-burning mechanism—metabolism—is a complex system of hormones and energy sources. It can be easily altered by too much stress and exercise, as well as too little sleep and food.

The focus on fat as bad is misplaced; rather, muscle is good. We are more concerned with the fat we can see than the hidden fat that is overproducing the hormones that regulate hunger and fat storage. We think that "fat-free" and "vegetarian" automatically makes something healthy and we lose track of the calories we consume when popping handfuls of nuts.

We confuse the sugar in soda with the sugar in an apple and forget that the fiber in fruits and vegetables makes a huge difference as far as our blood sugar level goes. And, did someone forget to mention what sugar has to do with fat anyway? Don't make these mistakes as you work to achieve your fat loss goals.

Misunderstanding Body Mass and Fat

Body Mass Index measures relative size based on the weight and height of an individual. In general, it quantifies a person's "thinness" or "thickness." A BMI of less than 18.5 is considered underweight, 18.5-25 normal weight, 25-30 overweight, and 30+ obese. However, for athletes and very active individuals, BMI does not accurately represent overall health as a high percentage of dense muscle mass and a low percentage of body fat also calculate as a high BMI (Dhillon).

Even the language of weight and fat perpetuates a misunderstanding of health and wellness. We give equal weight to skinny and fat, but there is no word opposite obesity. This hides some of the dangers that fat poses to individuals who are not overweight.

A thin person with little fat but also little muscle is worse off than obese individuals who are fit. In fact, Steven Blair, professor of exercise science, found that "obese individuals who are fit have a death rate one half that of normal-weight people who are not fit" (Katz).

A high metabolism and a genetic predisposition may keep someone thin but it is no guarantee against high blood pressure, cholesterol or blood sugar. A diet, not necessarily high in fat, but high in sugar and processed foods combined with inactivity will result in greater amounts of unseen visceral fat.

Cutting Calories

In an effort to lose fat, it can be tempting to skip meals and workout longer. After all, if you use more calories than you consume, losing fat should be as simple as just eating one less meal or doubling your morning jog. This, however, is the most common fat loss mistake. When under stress, the pituitary gland in the brain releases a hormone called adrenocorticotropic or ACTH.

The adrenal gland responds by producing a steroid hormone known as cortisol, which increases the body's ability to respond to the stressful situation, which in this case is self-induced. Skipping meals and extra exercise puts your body under undue stress. A small increase of cortisol results in a quick burst of energy, increased immunity, lower pain sensitivity, heightened memory function and general homeostasis in the body (Wisse).

So, you can work through your hunger until you eat again. However, cortisol also enlarges your fat cells and increases the amount of visceral fat in your body regardless of what you eat. While stress eating accounts for some of the weight gain, even those who respond to stress by not eating also retain fat because of this.

High and prolonged levels of cortisol is associated with high blood pressure, decreased bone density and muscle tissue, impaired cognitive performance, suppressed thyroid function, and lowered immunity and inflammatory responses (Scott). It also results in increased abdominal fat and thus heart attacks, strokes and metabolic syndrome. Not to mention a 10% decrease in body weight will slow metabolism to burn fewer calories and enhance the performance of muscle fibers in order to use less calories during exercise. The body will go to great lengths to defend the higher weight—for as many as six years.

Working Too Hard

Have you been waking up earlier to fit more workout sessions into your schedule? Not sleeping enough is associated with "a modest increase in future weight gain and incident obesity" (Patel). Regardless of exercise and diet, women who slept six hours gained weight and women who slept five hours or less gained even more.

These women were 30% more likely to gain belly fat than those who slept seven or more hours. Several hormones are at play when you don't get enough restful sleep. Cortisol levels are low and melatonin high at night when you go to sleep.

As you sleep, cortisol levels gradually increase throughout the night, naturally waking you in the morning. Leptin tracks the amount of fat stores available for potential energy, and it is only produced during certain stages of sleep. Ghrelin also induces hunger. Inadequate and interrupted sleep will disrupt cortisol, leptin and ghrelin levels.

Sleep has a noticeable effect on leptin and ghrelin levels in people who sleep only four hours a night. After just two days of sleep deprivation, they experience an 18% drop in leptin and 28% rise in ghrelin (Mercola). A drop in leptin signals a need to conserve fat stores and an increase in ghrelin signals hunger. Thus, regular and restful sleep is an important consideration in balancing the hormones that factor into fat loss.

Upping Cardio Exercise

This is a common mistake when it comes to exercise. To maintain a healthy weight, the Department of Health and Human Services recommends moderate or vigorous aerobic active three times a week and strength training exercises twice a week.

Four hours of cardiovascular exercise a week helped more than 40,000 women in their 40s and 50s lose weight in a 10-year study with the American Cancer Society (Kelly). It is important to be active regardless of size, meaning high intense aerobic activity as well as cardio and strength training.

Moderate activity will only slow weight gain and reduce the amount of visceral fat you gain. High intensity activity is what burns fat. However, even so, the body gets used to the activity and it becomes a less effective means of getting at fat reserves.

To avoid this plateau, alternate activities, work different muscle groups, integrate intervals of high intense activity—1 minute for every 3 minutes or even just 10 minutes a day. Full body workouts, combining strength training with cardio activity, build muscle as well. Remember any physical activity is an opportunity to burn calories and strengthen your body's muscles

Poor Nutrition

First off, do you know how many calories you eat in a day? Even worse, what calories are you drinking? Lattes and alcoholic beverages easily add calories to your day that your body stores as fat. Juice has all the sugar of fruit and vegetables with none of the fiber.

The sugar in juices and sodas is either burned instead of fat or stored directly as fat. And, the sweetness of zero calorie drinks confuses the brain causing cravings for more sugar and fat. Second, do you know what kind of calories you are eating?

Not all calories are made equal. 250 calories of sugar and fat is not the same as 250 calories of fiber and protein. Fat-loss takes consistent dedication to the right nutrition plan for your goals (Carneiro). Be wary of foods that you don't think of as fattening such as fat-free frozen yoghurt, peanut butter and bread that actually have added sugars that will not only spike your blood sugar level but add to the overproduction of insulin, the fat storage hormone, and leave you craving more sugar and fat.

Some super foods, while heavy hitters in omegas, micronutrients and phytogens, can be deceivingly small. Don't overeat when it comes to those almonds. And, even "vegetarian" diets can be unhealthy if you are eating more cheese and processed soy products than beans and vegetables.

While a no carbohydrate diet yields results in terms of weight, you may also feel sluggish and thick-headed. In the absence of carbohydrates, the body turns to alternate, though less optimum, energy sources including the body's own muscle mass and chemicals called ketones. Protein also will help you feel less hungry and therefore eat less throughout the day.

High-protein diets can have positive results on the body's blood lipids, glucose levels, and muscle-to-fat ratios. So, don't eliminate all carbohydrates, but balance 40% whole grains and fiber with 40% protein and 20% healthy fats. Yes, fat. While eating saturated fats common in meat and dairy leads to increased visceral fat, the healthy oils and monounsaturated fats found in olives, nuts and avocados have positive health effects on the body.

This includes building muscle mass, anti-inflammation, healthy cholesterol levels, at fat-soluble vitamins. Fat, like fiber and protein, also slows digestion and thus the absorption of sugar. This is especially important as simple sugars and processed foods result in blood sugar spikes that are draining, counterproductive to fat loss, and ultimately set the stage for decreased insulin sensitivity and type II diabetes. In general, a complete understanding of fat as well as a balanced approach to nutrition, exercise, and rest is essential to fat loss.

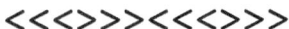

How to stop emotional eating and lose fat

Some people respond to stress by eating less and some people respond to stress by eating more. Surprisingly, one is not more common than the other. About the same amount of people overeat in response to stress as under eat with a few people unaffected. If you are one of those people who tend to pack on the pounds when stressed, the first step to fat loss is curbing emotional eating and recognizing the different triggers.

Emotional eating has several different triggers: negative thoughts, negative emotions, and social pressures. It can also be a symptom of atypical depression or a response to momentary or chronic stress. While emotional eating is fairly common, it is a significant factor in weight gain, obesity, and worse yet food addiction and bingeing and purging behaviors.

People who are susceptible to emotional eating also benefit more from stress reduction compared to people who eat less when exposed to stress. Thus, we can conclude that understanding and managing emotions and reducing stress is the best way to address emotional eating.

Emotional eating can be a symptom of atypical depression and binge eating

Not all emotional eating is related to depression or an eating disorder, however left unchecked it can perpetuate unhealthy eating habits. Comfort foods—ice cream, chocolate, cookies, chips, fries and pizza—are high-carbohydrate foods high in calories and often also sugar with little nutritional value.

Do you eat when you are bored or watching television? You may not know you are eating too much until it is too late and you have already put on extra belly fat. When in an emotional state, you may eat impulsively, too much, or whatever is convenient without thinking about it.

Have you been feeling sad or lonely? Your emotions become so entangled with your eating habits, that you become conditioned to eat when upset or stressed. Are you facing a difficult problem? Food can be a distraction if you are worried or avoiding dealing with conflict.

Emotional eating can suppress or soothe negative emotions caused by unemployment, financial pressure, health problems, relationship conflicts, work stress and fatigue. Regardless of the emotions momentarily suppressed, they eventually return, sometimes more than before spiraling into an unhealthy cycle. Basically, eating for comfort or any other reason than being physically hungry can become a problem.

Emotional eating can also be a symptom of other distinct and treatable mental illnesses including depression, atypical depression, binge eating disorder and bulimia. Most people with depression lose both energy and interest, in eating as well. However, feelings of worthlessness and sadness may result in emotional eating.

Atypical depression is a subset of depression. It differs in terms of mood reactivity, meaning that mood improves with positive events, and specific symptoms like increased appetite. People subject to chronic stress or abuse are at risk for chronically high levels of cortisol, which can lead to chronic emotional-eating patterns including increased appetite, craving comfort foods, and retaining belly fat.

In general, a few warning signs of emotional eating include suddenly feeling hunger intensely instead of gradually, craving junk food rather than balanced meals, wanting to eat in the face of uncomfortable emotions, and feeling guilty for eating.

Any psychological connection between food and comfort, power, reward or punishment can lead to emotional eating. Research suggests that girls and women are at higher risk for eating disorders and therefore, as a precursor, emotional eating. However, conflicting research has found that men are more likely than women to eat in response to depression or anger (Dryden-Edwards).

Recent research at UCLA explored how the brain reacts to negative emotions, food cravings and the reward center (Gupta). Bulimic women were shown a picture of a chocolate milkshake or water and given a taste of both. Their brain activity was monitored through use of an fMRI.

When a women with bulimia experiences negative emotions, the reward circuitry of her brain is more active in anticipation of food. Thus, the brain becomes conditioned to experience negative emotion as food cravings. Drinking the milkshake, however, does not register in the reward circuitry. They can keep eating and still not be satisfied. More research might show a similar function for any degree of overeating that is not related to physical need including depression and emotional eating.

You can be proactive in overcoming emotional eating

In overcoming emotional eating, it is important to disconnect food from feelings and associate food with sustenance. You have to learn (or re-learn) healthy ways to view food, develop better eating habits, recognize triggers, reduce stress, and develop appropriate coping strategies.

First, reframe your view of food. If you limit your calories too much and deprive yourself of all treats, cravings can actually intensify particularly in the context of emotional eating. If you are going to enjoy a treat, only eat what you love and eat it mindfully.

Don't feel guilty for it and don't eat it on an empty stomach. Director of the Recovery System Clinic, Julia Ross, explains, "If you've had a good meal with protein, vegetables, and a healthy fat, your dessert has a better chance of being emotionally satisfying" (Goad).

Saving calories in your meal and going straight for dessert will actually double up on the calories you skipped and cause a spike in blood sugar. Variety and the occasional treat will keep cravings at bay.

Check in with your eating habits and hold yourself accountable. In a food diary, record what you eat, how much, when and your emotional state. In this way, you can discover patterns and connections between food and mood specific to you.

"The more aware you are of your inner experiences, the more you can choose how to cope with them," psychologist Leslie Becker-Phelps says. If stress is a trigger, you can actively plan how to take control, change the situation, reframe your approach or thinking, or respond rather just reacting. And, if you fall into a bout of emotional eating, do not let it spiral out of control.

"Self-compassion is the first step toward learning to comfort yourself in other ways" (Manning). Focus on the positive changes and move forward learning from the experience. Once you understand your triggers, you can develop effective coping strategies for your emotional eating.

If stress is triggering your emotional eating, focus on stress management. Exercise! Regular physical activity decreases the production of stress chemicals which will help reduce depression, anxiety, insomnia and emotional eating. Or, meditate!

Meditation and other relaxation techniques are powerful tools in managing stress. Avoid drug and alcohol use. Many substances actually heighten the body's response to stress. Perhaps, boredom is a trigger. If you're bored, do something (just don't eat).

A short burst of activity, even walking in place for 10 minutes, will directly address stress and replace the urge to eat with something else. Go for a walk, watch a movie, pick up a book, listen to music, call a friend, or browse the internet. When craving food, double-check that you are actually hungry. If you ate recently and your stomach isn't rumbling, wait to see if the craving passes.

Telling yourself that you'll eat it later allows time for the impulse to pass and strengthens your sense of control. This delay also gives you time to check in with how you are feeling and the reasons you want to eat. Keep your hard-to-resist favorites out of sight or better yet don't stock them. If the food isn't there, you won't be tempted. If you still feel like a snack, choose a low-fat, low-calorie option.

Try some healthy foods that elevate mood

We eat because we are physically hungry, but sometimes we eat because we are sad, angry, stressed or bored. "We're hardwired to eat for emotional reasons," Dr. May says. "From the moment you're born and your mother holds you close to feed you, there's an emotional connection between being fed and being loved" (Goad).

Besides that the high calorie snacks we crave are packed with powerful natural chemicals that do elevate our mood. Caffeine makes you more alert; sugar results in a short-term burst of energy; and, chocolate contains serotonin and anandamide that interact with neurotransmitters to trigger a rush of endorphins that make you happy. However, you won't be able to avoid crashing after that sugar crash or caffeine buzz.

There are instead healthy alternatives that will positively influence your mood. A small amount, 200 mg, of caffeine will improve your mood but more than 24 ounces a day and the caffeine will do more harm than good. Make sure you're getting your recommended daily allowance of B-vitamins; try a bowl of fortified whole-grain cereal and banana.

Proteins like fish, eggs or lentils are high in tyrosine, an amino acid that boosts dopamine, a chemical that makes you feel good. Also, a vitamin D deficiency or low iron level will leave you feeling sluggish and tired, so eat your fruits, vegetables and fortified grains and get some sun.

Omega-3 fatty acids, folate, and selenium have also been found to have some beneficial effect for people with mild-to-moderate depression. Salmon, shrimp, lentils, bean salad, dark chocolate, fruit-yoghurt smoothies, and eggs will all leave you feeling better than before.

If after trying all of the suggestions described above, you should consider seeking professional help to control your emotional eating. A medical professional can check for physical causes of depression and weight gain, including hypothyroidism. And, a mental health provider can diagnose depression, anxiety, or an eating disorder.

Through therapy, you can understand the motivation and triggers of your emotional eating and develop coping skills and strategies. In particular, cognitive behavioral therapy (CBT) is an effective treatment for emotional eating. It sets up positive expectations for therapy, identifies the thoughts and assumptions that lead to emotional eating, and employs behavior-modification techniques (Dryden-Edwards).

Mindfulness increases your emotional awareness and reflective thinking so that you can separate your emotions from hunger. For those triggered by stress, stress-management counseling will help you develop not only stress-management skills but also support you in reducing stress. Nutritionists, therapists and support groups like Overeaters' Anonymous are all invaluable in developing healthy ways to approach food and recognize and cope with triggers.

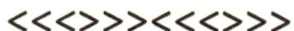

Eating habits for fat loss

How do people lose excess weight and keep it off? The National Weight Loss Registry gives us a small glimpse of what it takes. In general, almost all people, who have lost weight and kept it off, exercise on average an hour every day.

They simply stay more active, with 62% watching less than 10 hours of television a week. They constantly keep their weight maintenance in their minds: 75% weigh themselves at least once a week.

Now while there is also a wide range of how much weight lost and how long they have successfully kept off the weight, they also all have the same types of eating habits. They eat in a way that prevents weight gain. For example, 78% eat breakfast every day (http://www.nwcr.ws/research/). Successful weight control comes from small changes in your eating habits that add up to big calorie savings and weight loss.

Self-discipline begins with mastery over thought: who you are, and what you do. If you cannot control your thoughts, your actions are haphazard and unpredictable. This process requires self-knowledge and an accurate assessment of your current abilities. The source of all your failures and your successes lies in your habits. Even though we are creatures of habit, we can use the power of our minds to overcome our bodies and change our habits. This is true also of what you eat. Changing some of your basic eating habits will enable you to think first and eat afterward.

Daily Check-in

Start with an honest assessment of your eating habits. Are you nibbling while cooking or finishing off someone else's meal? Do you have a sweet tooth or struggle with junk food? Are you snacking when you're bored, lonely, or unhappy? Do you eat late at night? Developing strategies to deal with these feelings and temptations are half the battle. Ask for a takeout box.

Don't keep junk food in the house. Buy single serving packages of cookies. Treat your snacks like mini-meals; they should be high in complex carbohydrates with a little bit of protein and fat. Pack healthy snacks for the times when you know you are typically hungry. Make a menu plan for the week and use a shopping list to keep impulse buying to a minimum. And, never go to the grocery store when you're hungry.

You can allow yourself one indulgence purchase, but for the most part stick to your plan. And, track your calories. You can do this by hand or create a free account with one of the many health and fitness websites online.

Surprisingly, some of your best habits for fat loss start in the bathroom before you even start your day. Step on the scale at least once a day to keep track of the general range of what you weigh. Your weight will fluctuate daily, but you can catch small changes as they occur and track gradual weight loss.

If you weigh yourself in the morning, you'll weigh less than you do at night. People who also brush their teeth frequently are leaner. The minty-fresh flavor may help you snack less between meals. Good oral health care also prevents inflamed gums (periodontal disease). If your gums bleed when you floss, it is because they are sore and need help fighting the bacteria trying to sneak in every day through your mouth.

Research has found a correlation between high levels of inflammatory agents in the body and weight gain. So, brush your teeth 2-3 times a day after meals. If you want to savor the flavor of that cookie, just do a quick dry brush to knock that sugar off your teeth and prevent plaque buildup. Keep your gums healthy by flossing daily, rinsing with mouth wash, and making regular trips to the dentist.

Morning and Night

One of the most encouraging eating habits that will help you lose weight is just that: eating. Don't starve yourself and don't skip meals. Breakfast is the most important part of the day. It will kick start your metabolism and give you energy for the rest of the day. A good breakfast reduces hunger throughout the day and thus helps prevent overeating. You will make better food choices as well.

People who struggle with overeating are actually under eating during the first part of the day or skipping breakfast all together. Regular meals also help prevent bingeing. So, eat less more often. Charlene Johnson cites a study published in the New England Journal of Medicine: "When we go longer than 3 hours without eating, our levels of the stress hormone cortisol rise. And high cortisol levels signal the body to store fat in the abdominal region.

Keep in mind too that people who skip meals have the highest cortisol levels of all" (Johnson). Eating the same number of calories in six small meals rather than three large meals will reduce cortisol levels by more than 17%. By eating small, frequent meals, you are helping your body become more efficient at keeping cortisol levels low which will aid in fat loss.

Be aware of what you eat. Food is forgettable and unsatisfying when eaten out of packages and while standing. Fill up a small plate or take smaller portions and leave the extras back at the stove or in the fridge.

Drink water throughout the day and before meals. You should drink six to eight 12-ounce glasses plus more when exercising. Be careful not to drink too much water; more than a gallon of water a day will dilute the body of necessary electrolytes.

Eat slowly, drinking plenty of water with your meals. Take time to talk to other people when you're eating and give your body time to register that it's full. It can take up to 20 minutes. Eat an early dinner and don't eat anything afterwards.

If you're hungry have a non-caloric beverage or a piece of hard candy. Brushing your teeth after dinner also gives you a reason not to eat again. Never go to sleep on a full stomach. Digestion causes restless sleep and distracts the body from doing other important things. Going to bed earlier and without food needing to still be digested keeps your body's metabolism in a fat-burning state.

Know What You Are Eating

Become more knowledgeable about what you eat. Knowing how many calories, protein carbohydrate and fat is in the general foods that you eat will allow you to make better food choices on the spot. This isn't as hard as it sounds. After a couple weeks of reading labels will do the trick.

There are also phone apps and websites that will do this for you. Knowing what you like to eat, you can predict your daily calorie allotment and find foods that have what your body needs for energy and nutrition.

You don't have to go the extremes of planning every meal and researching every restaurant, but you can find healthy options on any menu. If your entrée comes with fries or a side of potatoes, ask for vegetables instead. You can politely request dressings and sauces on the side or little or no butter. Order your protein broiled, steamed, stir-fried or poached.

Avoid foods with high-fructose corn syrup. If you're going to eat something decadent, it's okay to be put on your foodie hat and turn up your nose and insist on real sugar and cream. The rise in sugar substitutes in the last four decades has paralleled an increase in obesity. Avoid processed carbohydrates including white flour and potatoes. "The calories from white bread and refined grains just seem to settle at the waistline more than calories from other foods" (Men's Fitness).

Potatoes, not including sweet potatoes which are higher in fiber and processed carbohydrates also raise the levels of insulin in the blood which signals the body to stop burning and start storing fat. This also leads to type 2 diabetes. Instead, fill up on whole foods—

fruits, vegetables and whole grains. Low density foods like apples, broccoli, brown rice and oatmeal are high in fiber and they will satisfy your hunger on fewer calories. High density foods—butter, oil, ice cream, candy—do the opposite.

The best eating habit for fat loss is that you can still eat your favorite foods...carefully. Denying yourself food that you love is setting yourself up for failure. The more you tell yourself you can't eat it, the more you think about it and the more you want it.

So, if you're going to eat ice cream or cake, take one scoop or a small slice. If you still want more, wait 20 minutes while your hormones kick in and satiate your cravings. It'll be easy to say no to a second serving after your brain has told your body that it is full.

If you follow a healthy diet 95% of the time, you can enjoy yourself the other 5% without gaining weight. In fact, if you eat more calories one day and fewer the next, your metabolism will stay active and keep burning fat at a high rate. In general, skipping meals, eating on the run and eating without thinking are the biggest eating habits you can change for fat loss. Enjoy food when you eat it, eat healthy food, weigh yourself, brush your teeth and get enough sleep.

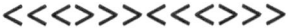

How to burn more belly fat

Every time you sit down, you can grab the stomach rolls by the handful. That skinfold you can pinch on your waist is not the belly fat that should worry you. Everyone has belly fat, even people with flat abs. Some of the fat is right under the skin, but the rest is inside the abdominal cavity cushioning the heart, lungs and other organs and is called visceral fat.

Too much of this fat can start to create buildups that are problematic for your health. As with all weight loss, a combination of a low-calorie diet high in fiber and low in sugar along with aerobic exercise and strength training is the best approaching to losing abdominal fat. You see it on your stomach so you think that sit-ups and crunches are going to melt the belly fat but spot training like this does not work.

Fortunately, when you lose weight on any diet, belly fat is the first to go. So, with healthy eating, aerobic activity, and exercise that targets your core muscles, the stomach flab will come off. More importantly you will seriously reduce the risk of developing type 2 diabetes, certain cancers, dementia and cardiovascular disease.

What is belly fat?

Adipose tissue, or body fat, consists of four kinds of fat: white, brown, subcutaneous and visceral fat. White fat are the fat cells that store energy and produce hormones that are secreted into the bloodstream.

The body relies on these fat cells as a necessary energy reserve. Brown fat actually burns calories to help regulate body temperature, but it makes up very little of the overall body fat. A person weighing 150 pounds might have 20-30 pounds of fat, of which 2-3 ounces will be brown fat. At its most efficient, those 2-3 ounces can burn 200-500 calories a day (Doheny). Children have more brown fat than adults, and lean people also have more brown fat than overweight or obese people. Additionally, brown fat declines with age.

Abdominal fat comes in two varieties: subcutaneous and visceral fat. The fat between the skin and the abdominal wall, as well as around the lower body, butt and thighs, is subcutaneous.

Belly fat is mostly visceral fat. Your genes determine how many fat cells you will develop and whether there are more in your mid-section or your lower body, making you pear or apple shaped.

Surgery can get at subcutaneous fat but Dr. Samuel Klein, professor of nutritional science at Washington University, found liposuction was an ineffective treatment for the "metabolic complications of obesity." Patients shed 30 pounds or more of subcutaneous fat through liposuction but they still had high blood pressure, cholesterol and blood sugar levels (Klein, 2004).

Is belly fat inevitable with age?

With age, the body's metabolism and ability to burn calories changes as well as how it stores and uses fat. Metabolism slows down, so the number of calories the body needs decreases. Likewise, muscle burns fat and so loss of muscle mass with age decreases how fast the body uses its available energy.

Overall, muscle loss contributes to an unfavorable shift in the proportion of fat to body weight, for both men and women. However, for women, the ratio of fat-to-lean tissue and fat storage begins to favor the stomach area over the hips and thighs.

Women, in particular, will gain belly fat even if they aren't gaining weight. Even women who don't gain weight during menopause still find that their waistline increases. Production of estrogen and progesterone slows during menopause.

Testosterone levels also drop but at a slower rate. Estrogen levels influence fat distribution throughout the body. When women gain weight after menopause, they carry it around the waist instead of on their hips and thighs. This shift in hormone levels causes women to carry more weight in their bellies transforming the body from a "pear" to an "apple" shape.

How much belly fat do you have?

Visceral fat can only be exactly determined through a CT scan or MRI, however BMI, waist-to-hip ratio, and waist circumference are commonly used. The waist circumference is the most common measurement of abdominal fat because it is just as accurate, even easier, to measure than waist-to-hip ratio.

It also indicates fat distribution whereas the body mass index indicates only total body fat. To measure belly fat, wrap a tape measure around your bare stomach, at your belly button, just above your hipbone. Resist the urge to suck in your stomach. A waist measurement of more than 35 in (89 cm) for women and 40 in (102 cm) for men is an unhealthy concentration of belly fat.

A "pear" shape with bigger hips and thighs is safer than an "apple" shape with a wider waistline. "What we're really pointing to with the apple versus pear," Kristen Hairston, MD says, "is that, if you have more abdominal fat, it's probably an indicator that you have more visceral fat" (Collins).

Why is belly fat worse than thigh fat?

Fat serves a dual purpose in the body. It safely stores excess calories as well as releases hormones that control metabolism. Fat cells, especially abdominal fat cells, are biologically active producing "lots of nasty substances" (Collins).

As an endocrine organ, or gland, too much fat can lead to a metabolic syndrome –high blood pressure, high blood sugar levels, excess abdominal fat, and abnormal cholesterol levels—which is a major risk factor of heart disease and stroke.

Fat cells also produce the stress hormones, cortisol, and inflammatory substances, like cytokines, that regulate metabolism and the immune system. Excess fat cells produce so much of the hormone leptin that reduces hungry that the body begins to resist it and they produce less of the hormone adiponectin that makes the body sensitive to insulin.

Fat cells produce leptin that suppresses appetite and regulates ghrelin, another hormone that signals hunger and cravings to the brain (Magee). While high levels of fat obviously results in more leptin, people develop a resistance to the appetite-cutting effects of leptin and do no register that there is plenty of body fat available as an energy resource.

Besides appetite regulation, leptin also plays a role in learning and memory. The increased levels of leptin may have an adverse effect on the brain leading to dementia. Adiponectin, produced by fat cells, makes the liver and muscles sensitive to insulin. However, the body produces less adiponectin as belly fat increase. Thus, increased body fat negatively affects the body's production of insulin increasing the risk for type 2 diabetes.

Cytokines also increase the risk of cardiovascular disease by promoting low-level chronic inflammation, increasing blood pressure and affecting blood clotting. It's safe to say that too much belly fat upsets the normal balance and function of these hormones.

There's only so much space in the abdominal cavity. If the regular areas to store fat are all at capacity, weight gain finds its way into some unusual places. Your body will start to store fat around the heart and even in vital organs.

Your body starts storing white fat in and around your heart, lungs, and liver, instead of just cushioning these very essential organs. As visceral fat builds up around the liver, it releases substances, including free fatty acids, into the blood through the portal vein that carries blood from the intestines to the liver.

This affects the production of blood lipids. Visceral fat is directly linked to high overall cholesterol, high LDL (bad) cholesterol and low HDL (good) cholesterol. According to Harvard Health, studies have found that a waist-to-hip ratio over 0.85 for women is associated with a 52% increase in colorectal cancer risk.

People with a higher waist-to-hip ratio experience equal difficulty with various daily activities as people with a high Body Mass Index despite being within a normal weight range. A large waist measurement, regardless of total body fat, meaning if you have more belly fat than anywhere else, is also a predictor for the development of high blood pressure.

Combine aerobic exercise and strength training

Even thin people, if they are do not exercise enough; can have too much visceral fat. It's important to be active regardless of size, meaning high intense aerobic activity as well as cardio and strength training.

You should get 30-60 minutes of moderate exercise, which raises the heart rate, causes you to breathe harder and work up a sweat, at least five days a week. However, moderate activity will only slow weight gain and reduce the amount of visceral fat you gain.

High intensity activity is what burns fat. Instead of walking five times a week for 30 minutes each time, go jogging four times a week for 20 minutes each time. Set the treadmill for a slight incline or use the stationary bikes, elliptical and rowing machines.

Do some yard work, play soccer, or go to Zumba. Raking leaves can be high intensity exercise; you don't have to work out at the gym. You can also stand in place and do squats here is a link on how to do them properly: https://www.youtube.com/watch?v=UXJrBgI2RxA the faster you go doing these types of squats the more fat you will burn.

Visceral fat does respond to the same diet and exercise strategies recommended for overall fat loss. However, it comes off more easily with aerobic exercise – running, biking, or swimming – rather than resistance training.

Running the equivalent of 12 miles a week should do the trick. Researchers at Duke University Medical Center found that the non-exercisers experienced a nearly 9% gain in visceral fat after six months. Subjects who exercised the equivalent of walking or jogging 12 miles per week put on no visceral fat, and those who exercised the equivalent of jogging 20 miles per week lost both visceral and subcutaneous fat.

A cardio workout alone isn't enough. Strength training (exercising with weights) may also help fight abdominal fat. A University of Pennsylvania study followed overweight or obese women, ages 24–44, for two years.

Those who did weight training twice a week reduced their proportion of body fat by nearly 4%. Strength training increases muscle mass and "muscle burns more calories than fat, and therefore you naturally burn more calories throughout the day by having more muscle" (Rossi).

Kate Patton, registered dietician, recommends 4 hours of moderate-intensity exercise or 2 hours of high-intensity exercise a week. Low-intensity workouts result in very little fat loss. Personal trainers stress exercising "at full intensity because the end goal is to burn more calories and high intensity exercise does just that" (Rossi). High intensity workouts mean you're going all out for as long as you can.

In short, depending on your age and genetic risk, you may be more pear shaped or more apple shaped. However, regardless of your size, it is important to stay active. Too much visceral fat can upset the body's hormonal balance affecting metabolism, memory, blood sugar and cholesterol levels. This increases the risk of several cancers, dementia, diabetes and heart disease. It can also encroach on vital organs.

Even thin people can have too much visceral fat. Aerobic exercise, moderate to high intense activity, will evenly use all of the body's fat but belly fat tends to go first. Strength training and exercises that work the core abdominal muscles will tone muscle but it will also build more muscle, and muscle burns more calories than fat does.

Embrace your weight

Despite the clear-cut formula of the Body Mass Index, weight is not synonymous with fat, no more than fat is synonymous with ugly, lazy or unhealthy. Adipose tissue not only stores fat but it is an important endocrine and secretory organ essential in metabolism.

Fat also cushions and protects our internal organs, coats our nerves, conserves heat, and regulates female menstruation. It is just as important to have healthy fat as it is to have a healthy heart, liver or lungs.

Many hormones can disrupt the healthy balance of our fat, including leptin, ghrelin, insulin, and cortisol. While healthy eating habits will balance hunger and fat storage hormones and sleep and exercise are beneficial to reducing levels of stress hormones, part of reducing stress comes from embracing your weight.

Above all, the plethora of mixed cultural messages about fat can wreak havoc with your health goals. What does it mean to be overweight? Are you fat and at risk for all the dangers associated with obesity? Is it better to be underweight even if that means losing some voluptuous curves or muscle mass?

If you have an apple rather than a pear shape, gain weight easily or have a slow metabolism, losing weight can be difficult. Your activity and diet could have also been disrupted by surgery or restricted due to a disability.

Weight gain or loss is also a side effect of some medications. But, even skinny people can be at risk for diabetes, heart diseases, and infertility if they have too much hidden fat or not enough fat.

Embracing your weight is the healthiest way to maintain your target weight and an overall healthy lifestyle.

In our effort to be healthy and fit, we must also keep in mind cultural misconceptions of what fat is and what it means. People come in all shapes and sizes, but so often we focus on the numeric clothing size. A size 2 isn't too skinny if you're 5 feet tall, and 155 pounds isn't overweight if you're a triathlete. In fact, what is classified as overweight looks fairly normal as seen in Kate Harding's Shapely Prose project (Harding).

Some therapists, scientists and others have supported a "fat acceptance" philosophy in order to focus on improving physical and mental health while stabilizing weight. This fat acceptance has made its way into the mainstream with outspoken celebrities, models and athletes like Oprah Winfrey and tennis player Monica Sales who had to "throw out the word 'diet'" to be healthy and strong.

Crystal Renn's modeling career took off when she became a "plus-size" model. At a size 12, and now a size 10 after hiking and yoga, she's hardly a "plus-size" model. Culturally, we associate fat with obesity and a list of negative personal characteristics like lazy, ugly, stupid, and undisciplined.

It is important to remember that muscle weighs more than fat and weight loss is not as important as fat loss, particularly visceral fat. While BMI can be one indicator of health, we should be mindful that the formula does not work in every situation.

While we have a word for fat and skinny, overweight and underweight, there is no parallel word for obese or morbidly obese. This is less a product of science a more indicative of a cultural bias and erasure of the dangers of being underweight. The truth is that even skinny people can be fat and unhealthy. In general, regardless of weight, it is important to develop an active and fun lifestyle and healthy eating habits that is mindful of blood sugar levels.

The obvious downside to being underweight is not having enough fat. Low body fat contributes to amenorrhea, disrupted menstruation and irregular periods. It also affects fertility.

Weight loss correlates with a drop in the female sex hormone estrogen and so being thin can make it difficult to get pregnant. However, that's not the only factor contributing to fertility. With IVF treatment, we see that thin women produce the same number of eggs as overweight women. However, the embryos are less likely to attach and implant in very thin women.

Dr. Richard Sherbahn looked at data from 2,500 sessions of IVF over eight years at the Advanced Fertility Center of Chicago. 45% of obese women, including those considered dangerously obese, and 50% of the normal weight women conceived and had babies, while only 34% of women considered very thin had babies.

In the UK, hospitals will actually refuse to fund IVF treatment for women who are underweight (Macrae). In any case, a woman has a greater chance of getting pregnant if she is close to her ideal weight, but she has less of a chance if she is under rather than over her ideal body weight.

The less obvious danger in being underweight is that a skinny person might still have too much fat. A high metabolism and a genetic predisposition make keep someone thin but it is no guarantee against high blood pressure, cholesterol or blood sugar. A diet, not necessarily high in fat, but high in sugar and processed foods combined with inactivity will result in greater amounts of visceral fat, which unlike subcutaneous fat is not visually apparent.

Fat is an obvious indicator of health, but visceral fat unlike subcutaneous fat (the fat directly under the skin) is embedded within your abdominal cavity, cushioning your vital organs and sometimes encroaching on your heart, lungs and liver.

Visceral fat likes inactivity, and people who diet but don't exercise are still likely to have too much visceral fat. High levels of visceral fat can cause metabolic syndrome including several conditions like high blood pressure and high blood sugar that put them at risk for diabetes, heart disease and stroke.

Daniel Neides, medical director at Cleveland Clinic's Wellness Institute says, "On the outside, they look incredibly healthy, but on the inside, they're a wreck" (Sifferlin). High levels of body fat, regardless of BMI, are still at risk for cardiovascular disease and a significantly higher risk of metabolic problems than other groups.

One out of four adults with a normal weight has high blood pressure or cholesterol in the U.S. Being too thin, like extreme obesity, is equally correlated with higher mortality rates. People at high risk for developing diabetes, including skinny and fat people, will best prevent the disease by eating a healthy diet, exercising, managing stress and abstaining from smoking.

Fluctuating weight or weight cycling also leads to overall belly fat and weight gain and the same medical conditions attributed to obesity. In 2005, nutrition professor Linda Bacon, who coined the term Health at Every Size, compared women who dieted and women instructed in HAES.

She found that while neither group lost weight, the HAES participants were healthier and more physically active with higher self-esteem. The basic public health belief continues to be that is dangerous to be fat.

As Walter Willett, chairman of the nutrition department at the Harvard School of Public Health, puts it: "Virtually everyone who is overweight would be better off at a lower weight...the data are clear" (Katz). There is still no agreement on the best or even a possible way to keep weight off long-term for the majority of people. But, everyone agrees that regular exercise and healthy eating habits improves health.

The research of Steven Blair, professor of exercise science, epidemiology and biostatistics, indicates that "obese individuals who are fit have a death rate one half that of normal-weight people who are not fit" (Katz). Dieting doesn't always lead to permanent weight loss, but neither does giving up dieting. For some ex-dieters, intuitive-eating does result in slimming down, but others just end up where they started. It is more important that weight loss not be used a placeholder for more important dreams and ambitions.

When you do reach your target weight, you will face many of the mental challenges of weight loss including self-doubt, frustration, and general discouragement. It is important to embrace your new body or you risk undermining your accomplishments and efforts.

If excess weight had previously been a defense mechanism or emotional eating a coping strategy, address those emotional issues in positive ways by finding healthy ways to deal with difficult emotions or taking steps to confront and resolves the issue (Pearson).

Support groups and therapy are also responsible and appropriate strategies when talking a walk or making a list doesn't seem to be enough. Don't continue to think of yourself as a "fat" person. Letting go of limiting beliefs is why HAES works.

Replace assumptions about tasteless healthy food or the inevitability of weight gain with empowering beliefs that help you maintain your weight and healthy habits. Be mindful not to fall back into old habits.

Don't deny yourself an occasional treat but don't stock up on sweets or skip regular workouts. Remember you don't have to do it all alone but be prepared for a variety of reactions from others, well-meaning and otherwise. An objective counselor can help you develop the flexibility, fortitude and coping skills necessary to maintain your new weight.

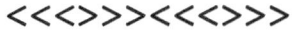

How to lose fat by eating more

Losing fat should be as simple as not eating, especially in today's fast-paced life where it is easy to skip breakfast or work through lunch and pass on midmorning or afternoon snacks. However, to lose fat and keep it off, this is not enough.

You can lose weight by restricting calories and eating less but your body will fight you tooth and nail for every calorie lost. After long periods of not eating, your body falls into a catabolic state where it starts to break down muscle tissue instead of fat. It starts dropping muscle rather than burn into its fat reserves, and it becomes ever more efficient requiring fewer and fewer calories to maintain its weight.

It'll even drive you crazy, as hormones start making you feel hungrier and making fatty foods even more irresistible. Losing fat isn't about not eating; it's about what you eat. And, what you can eat, you can lose fat by eating more of it. When it comes to losing fat, you do not need to work harder—exercising and dieting more. Rather, you will lose fat by working smarter—eating regularly, eating high volume and low calorie snacks, and eating enough to reduce craving.

Never skip breakfast

Before starting your day, eat breakfast combining protein and carbohydrates. The worst breakfast is no breakfast at all. When it comes to burning fat, it really is the most important meal of the day. Breakfast jump starts your metabolism and gives you energy for the day.

If you don't eat in the morning, your metabolism slows. As fat cells shrink, they secrete less leptin which the brain senses and responds by increasing hunger and decreasing your metabolic rate. This leads to poor food choices later in the day being processed more slowly.

Harvard and Boston's Children's Hospital found that obesity rates are 35%-50% lower in people who eat breakfast regularly compared to those who often skip this meal. You should be getting a third of your daily calories early in the day. Regularly skipping breakfast, results in a 450% increase in risk for obesity (Men's Fitness). Breakfast also helps regulate insulin levels and hunger, so you're less likely to overeat throughout the remainder of the day.

If you aren't feeling hungry, drink a glass of lemon water or eat something small like fruit and toast. This will stimulate your mind and body and stir your appetite. If you don't have time or desire for a large breakfast, eat like a hobbit.

Have a small breakfast first and then eat a light mid-morning meal, common in other countries as a second breakfast. Drink a glass of 1% milk which is 8 grams of protein plus fat-burning calcium. Or, eat some cereal and then grab fruit and a yogurt later to eat at work. A small breakfast will give you energy and help you focus throughout the day. Eggs and toast has always been a good breakfast option: toast and egg with tomato slices; tofu scramble with cheese; whole grain toast with almond butter and banana; and, scrambled eggs, broccoli, chicken and feta in a whole grain pita.

Other traditional breakfast options include: yogurt or cottage cheese with fresh fruit topped with nuts, seed and ground flaxseed; oatmeal or quinoa with apples, cinnamon and pecans; and, smoothies made with fruit, yogurt and soy milk. Leftovers also work: sliced lean meat or cheese and tomato; tuna salad with cheese and a pickle; and, leftover chili, stir fry, chicken or paella. Whether small or large, breakfast must include protein, grains, and veggies or fruit.

Eat more snacks and meals

While you will lose weight by skipping meals and eating fewer calories, you will also gain it back. The best way to lose weight is to protect your muscles and fuel your metabolism so it stays high. Eating less but more frequently will help keep your energy levels constant and your metabolism active. Regular meals and snacks also help prevent bingeing and overeating. So, eat less more often.

You can reduce cortisol levels by more than 17% by dividing your daily calories over six small meals, rather than three large meals. Chalene Johnson cites a study published in the New England Journal of Medicine: "When we go longer than 3 hours without eating, our levels of the stress hormone cortisol rise. And high cortisol levels signal the body to store fat" (Johnson).

By eating small, frequent meals, you are helping your body become more efficient at keeping cortisol levels low which will aid in fat loss.

To keep your portions small at meal times, drink a glass of water or start with a side salad or vegetable-only appetizer. To create a low calorie but balanced meal, fill half of your plate with colorful fruits and vegetables, a quarter with grains, potatoes or legumes, and a quarter of higher calorie protein-rich food. You can cut your entrée in half and substitute it with soup or salad.

Instead of snacking on crackers and cheese or other processed foods, try popcorn, peanuts, or apple slices. Small meals like soups, sandwiches, sushi and leftovers are all good choices. Choose snacks like vegetable sticks, fruit, nuts, hummus and yogurt dip over juice, muffins and other snacks high in sugar or fat. If you fill your plate with high volume, low calorie and nutrient dense foods, you will fuel your metabolism and satiate your hunger pangs.

Treat yourself and reduce cravings

In order to fill up your stomach without overloading on calories, fill up on some low calorie snacks. Snacking will help prevent overeating at meals, and it also keeps your body processing food all day long keeping your metabolism active throughout the day.

Having prepared snacks will also help cut snacking on candy or chips from the vending machine. In order to fill up your stomach without overloading on calories, fill up on these low calorie snacks. Fruits, vegetables, soups and oatmeal are 80-95% water so they are naturally lower in calories (Zelman).

Oatmeal is more filling than dry cereal with the same amount of calories and fiber. Two cups of grapes has the same amount of calories as ¼ cup of raisins but it takes longer to eat. Some other high volume, low calorie snacks that you could enjoy include: dill pickles, cherry tomatoes, bell peppers and hummus, and frozen vegetables and fruit. In general, adding more fruit and vegetables to your diet increases the amount of food you eat while simultaneously decreasing the total number of calories consumed.

While healthy but high-calorie snacks such as nuts and dried fruits should only be consumed in small amounts, nuts will make you feel full more so than other foods. University of Michigan researchers found that adding nuts to your diet does not result in additional weight (Men's Fitness).

So, you can fill a small snack baggie with dried blueberries, walnuts and high fiber cereal like bran flakes. Or, you can enjoy a nice granola bar made with real nuts and whole grains knowing that it is high in fiber and protein. You can also dress up your apple with some chopped nuts or a tablespoon of nut butters, or you can trade out your potato chips for soy chips which are also high in protein and low in calories.

Because fat has twice as many calories as protein or carbohydrates, reducing the amount of fat is one of the most efficient ways to take in fewer calories without having to give up your favorite foods. You can satisfy cravings and cut calories by choosing the low fat options of your most favorite treats: sorbet, frozen yogurt, light ice cream and fruit based desserts.

Research suggests that calcium helps the body burn fat. Portion-controlled snacks, like fig newton snack packs and novelty ice cream bars, will also satisfy your sweet tooth without blowing all your calories on one treat. If you like candy, have a handful of licorice. Real licorice, high in licorice extract, contains glycrrhetinic acid, an ingredient that blocks an enzyme that plays a role in fat accumulation (Women's Health). The sweetness will also quiet those cravings for more.

At the end of the day, if you eat more in the right ways, you will lose fat. Eat a good breakfast, several small meals throughout the day, snack on high-fiber and protein combos, and soothe your sweet tooth with low-fat treats. Have a big breakfast or two small breakfasts, so long as you frontload on your daily calories and then eat again every 3-5 hours. Fill up on high volume snacks: grapes, air popped popcorn and pickles.

Remember, nuts are rich in protein and the extra calories actually do not result in extra weight. Likewise, research shows that the calcium in some of your favorite low-fat treats like yogurt and ice cream also burns fat. Even something sweet like licorice will help fight fat accumulation. By eating more of the right kinds of food, you will turn the tide in your body's war against fat.

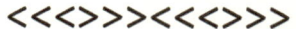

The ultimate fat loss secret

While some foods more than others will help or hinder weight loss, the secret to fat loss is still: burn more calories than you consume. Weight overall is the result of the balance of the calories you eat and the energy you burn. If you eat more than you exercise, you will store the extra calories as fat. Even if you eat little but do not exercise, you will not build muscle and your metabolism may even drop in an effort to conserve energy reserves holding on to the weight that you do have.

Age also complicates the body's ability to hold on to muscles decreasing the rate at which the body uses calories. Until scientists discover the perfect cocktail for weight loss, more than anything else, including reducing calories, exercise will help you maintain a healthy weight through sustainable weight loss.

Depending on your age and genetic risk, you may be more pear shaped or more apple shaped. However, regardless of your size, it is important to stay active. Too much visceral fat can upset the body's hormonal balance affecting metabolism, memory, blood sugar and cholesterol levels. This increases the risk of several cancers, dementia, diabetes and heart disease (Harvard Health). It can also encroach on vital organs.

Even thin people can have too much visceral fat. Aerobic exercise, moderate to high intense activity, will evenly use all of the body's fat but belly fat tends to go first. Strength training and exercises that work the core abdominal muscles will tone muscle but it will also build more muscle, and muscle burns more calories than fat does. Regardless of size, aerobic exercise and strength training is the ultimate secret to fat loss.

Fidgeting burns calories

Small changes in your everyday routine will build in more activity and energy use. Research shows that there is a connection between sleep and a healthy metabolism, so skip the late night comedy shows and get a little bit more sleep. Take a look at the number of hours you spend sitting in front of a computer or watching television or video clips online. This sedentary lifestyle is weighing you down, literally.

Researchers at the Mayo Clinic found that sedentary individuals gain eight times more weight than those who fidget a lot (Men's Fitness). Fast forward through the commercials or better yet just get off the couch. If you need a little bit of extra motivation, watch a movie that inspires you to exercise like Rocky or Without Limits. Joining a sports league will also build in vigorous exercise into your week and the team motivation will keep you showing up.

Individuals on the National Weight Control Registry, who have successful lost and kept weight off, weigh themselves every day. Rena Wing, Ph.D., founder of the registry, explains why this is important: "keep track of the general range of what you weigh so you can catch small changes as they occur and take corrective measures immediately" (Men's Fitness).

This also gives you a sense of control over your weight and a reason to keep up the effort. Any kind of physical activity is good. You will burn fat by raking the leaves, mowing the lawn or cleaning out the gutters. Sneak extra activity into your day by walking or biking to do errands. Stop using the drive-thru, and pace or stand when you could be sitting. Take the stairs instead of the elevator and skip one out of every five steps. And, to help you keep it in the forefront of your mind, step on the scale once a day.

Beef up your workout routine

Just 10 minutes a day, three days a week, of weight training before working out will help lose the fat faster. A cardio workout, with the same speed and intensity, after weight lifting will have a greater affect than if you had just gone running. Workout standing up— you will use up to 30% more calories just by standing instead of sitting.

Make your work out more efficient by alternating between lower body exercises and upper body exercises. Close your eyes while you exercise so that the core muscles have to work harder to keep you balanced. Try to outdo yourself and break your own records, even if you only challenge yourself to run one-tenth of a mile more in the same amount of time as the workout before.

If you are running on a treadmill, make sure that you walk or run on at least a 1% incline to equalize the force that you normally get from running outside. Changing directions also boosts your body's fat-burning efforts because of the force required to stop your momentum and reverse the moment at full speed.

Burn fat by building muscle

Don't think that you can trim the fat by doing a bunch of sit ups every day. Targeted abdominal exercises like crunches or sit-ups will tone abdominal muscles and provide definition, but it will not get rid of belly fat. Spot exercising, such as sit-ups, can tighten abdominal muscles, but it does not help decrease the visceral fat in your abdominal cavity. Abdominals include the many interconnected muscles that run up the back and stretch down to the butt and the front and inner thighs.

So, you should focus on strength training that exercises your entire core. Instead, focus on functional exercises that use the muscles in your core—abdominals, back, pelvic, obliques—as well as other body parts. These exercises use more muscles, so there is a higher rate of calorie burn.

Plank exercises activate not just your core muscles but also your arm, leg, and butt muscles. Engage the core, tightening all of the muscles, keeping hips parallel to the floor and moving from the waist. For any strength training exercise, exhale deeply.

Consistent and deep breathing will strengthen your core muscles and protect your lower back. Other variations of plank exercises, like side plank engage your core even more as you stack your legs and lift your hips to form a straight line from head to feet. This also works your triceps, biceps, core, and waist.

Or, try a swan dive, lying on your stomach. Keeping your arms straight along your body, arch your back and legs up. Of course, work up to more challenging poses. Don't go straight into side plank. Do some swan dives and plank exercises, before going into a side plank position. Drop a knee if you need too. Hold each position for 8th breaths.

Try a variety of crunch exercises: cross your legs and hold them in the air for each crunch. Cross over in a diagonal crunch. Pull your legs in for leg crunches or lift them and circle each leg in the air one at a time. Move your knees from side to side like windshield wipers. Or, try some standing side crunches.

Whatever you do on one-side of the body, make sure to work the other side. Donkey kickbacks are a killer move that will burn calories and work the core muscles. Kneel on all fours, toes tucked under, keeping your back neutral. Draw your belly in toward your spine as you contract your abs and kick back.

You can also use your own body weight to work your core as you do repeated squats, or hold a sitting position and push off the floor with your arms. This is not only good for the core and arm muscles but it also strengthens the pelvic floor.

A variety of boat poses will also target abdominal muscles without the uncomfortable friction of sitting up. Sit with your feet on the floor, knees bent, hands beneath your knees for support. Keeping your chest lifted and shoulders back, engage your abdominal muscles and raise your lower legs until they are parallel to the floor. Work up to each position, keeping your knees bent at first and balancing on your sitting bones. Hold the pose for 8 breaths. You can build up to a full boat pose by stretching out one leg at a time and releasing your hold on your legs until both legs are held in the air with free arms out stretched. To use your fast-twitch muscle fibers (the ones that contract during high-intensity moves and improve muscle tone) sit up into this v-position quickly three times.

To maintain a healthy weight, you must eat a healthy diet in small portions and include physical activity in your daily routine. Your diet should be high in fiber and protein and low in saturated fats and sugar. Too much weight loss at once will negatively alter the body's metabolism, so gradual weight loss –2 pounds a week – will help to keep the excess fat from coming back.

To maintain a healthy weight, the Department of Health and Human Services recommends strength training exercises twice a week and moderate aerobic activity like brisk walking (at least 150 minutes) or vigorous aerobic activity like jogging (at least 75 minutes) (Mayo Clinic). To lose weight, you will have to exercise more than that. Remember any physical activity is an opportunity to burn calories and strengthen your body's muscles.

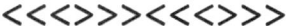

How to obey the rules of fat loss

After careful consideration, we have identified the laws of fat burning. In order to burn energy at an optimum level for fat loss, we must keep the body's metabolism active, maintain even blood sugar and hormone levels, and build muscle. However, keeping these laws of fat burning is more complicated than just using more calories than consumed.

The body takes precautionary measures against losing too much weight conserving fat reserves and craving fatty foods until you have gained back the weight. It can be difficult not to spike your blood sugar levels, when sugar seems to be in everything and everyday life continues to be stressful.

As challenging as fat loss is, a holistic approach of healthy eating, balanced exercise, reasonable relaxation, and a positive and patient mental attitude will lead to steady improvements in your overall lifestyle, health, and, along with that, fat loss.

Healthy Eating

Healthy eating involves when and how much you eat, what you eat and what you don't eat. Skipping meals does more harm than good when it comes to your metabolism. Aim to eat organic foods that are high in fiber and protein and avoid processed foods with added sugar and food additives. Excitotoxins end up in our processed foods as food additives and derivatives as well as on our fresh produce from chemicals sprays, dips and baths. While they make the food tasty, it also turns off our natural sense of satiety, so we keep eating until the bag is empty.

Food additives are often allergenic causing insulin to spike adding to pre-diabetes factors (Salerno). And, last, the chemicals that help keep our produce without blemish also increase food cravings, water retention and weight gain.

Become more knowledgeable about what you eat. Knowing how many calories, protein carbohydrate, sugar and fat is in the general foods that you eat will allow you to make better food choices on the spot. Avoid foods with high-fructose corn syrup and other refined sugars.

A Princeton University study found that rats gained significantly more weight consuming the same amount of calories from HFCS as with table sugar. It also led to a larger increase in belly fat and circulating triglycerides (Kamb).

Besides sugar content, processed foods have the same effect on blood sugar level as glucose. Potatoes, not including sweet potatoes, and processed carbohydrates also raise the levels of insulin in the blood which signals the body to stop burning and start storing fat.

Instead, fill up on whole foods—fruits, vegetables and whole grains; the fiber slows digestion and thus affects blood sugar levels more gradually. Low density foods like apples, broccoli, brown rice and oatmeal are high in fiber and they will satisfy your hunger on fewer calories. High density foods—butter, oil, ice cream, candy— do the opposite.

Regular Eating

When it comes to burning fat, breakfast is the most important meal of the day. Breakfast jump starts your metabolism and gives you energy for the day. In fact, if you don't eat in the morning, your metabolism slows.

As fat cells shrink, they secrete less leptin which the brain senses and responds by increasing hunger and decreasing your metabolic rate. This leads to poor food choices later in the day being processed more slowly.

You should be getting a third of your daily calories early in the day. If you aren't feeling hungry, drink a glass of lemon water or eat something small like fruit and toast to stimulate your mind and body and stir your appetite. Or, have a small breakfast and then a light mid-morning meal to give you energy and help you focus throughout the day. Whether small or large, breakfast must include protein, grains, and veggies or fruit.

While you will lose weight by skipping meals and eating fewer calories, you will also gain it back. If you go longer than three hours without eating, levels of the stress hormone cortisol increase which signal the body to store fat.

You can reduce cortisol levels by more than 17% by dividing your daily calories over six small meals, rather than three large meals (Johnson). Eating less but more frequently will help keep your energy levels constant and your metabolism active.

Regular meals and snacks also help prevent bingeing and overeating. Keep your portions small at meal times by starting with a glass of water or a vegetable-only appetizer and then balancing half of the meal with fruits and vegetables and split the other half between whole grains and protein.

Choose snacks like vegetable sticks, fruit, nuts, hummus and yogurt dip rather than juice, muffins and other snacks high in sugar or fat. If you fill your plate with high volume, low calorie and nutrient dense foods, you will fuel your metabolism and satiate your hunger pangs.

Cardio, Strength and Interval Training

Fat loss results from a balance between cardiovascular exercises; strengthen training, full body workouts and interval training. Excessive cardio to the exclusion of other types of exercise will actually result in muscle efficiency to perform by burning fewer calories. However, regular cardio exercise is still important for your overall fitness and visceral fat appears to come off more easily with aerobic exercise.

Subjects in a study at Duke University Medical Center who exercised the equivalent of walking or jogging 12 miles per week put on no visceral fat, and those who exercised the equivalent of jogging 20 miles per week lost both visceral and subcutaneous fat.

The non-exercisers experienced a nearly 9% gain in visceral fat after six months. Strength training also helps fight abdominal fat as it increases muscle mass and muscle burns more calories than fat. A University of Pennsylvania study found that women who did weight training twice a week reduced their proportion of body fat by nearly 4%. Kate Patton, registered dietician, recommends 4 hours of moderate-intensity exercise or 2 hours of high-intensity exercise a week (Rossi).

Interval training is a type of cardiovascular exercise that builds muscle mass and boosts your metabolism as well as strengthens the heart. It involves a short period of exercises that requires a high level of exertion, usually a weight-bearing cardiovascular exercise that uses large groups of muscle and requires the body to work very hard to supply enough energy.

This is then followed by an exercise that requires a lower level of exertion. The benefits of interval training include improved cardiovascular fitness, increased stamina and thus better athletic performance, but also fat loss and more muscle mass, and thus a higher metabolism.

Try a 30-60-90 workout of five cycles: 30 seconds hard and easy, then 60 seconds, and 90 seconds repeating four times. A 3 on 1 off workout is four cycles of 3 minutes of moderate intensity and 1 minute at high intensity (Mirlenbrink). Both include appropriate time to warm up and cool down, always mindful of signs that your body has had enough. Interval workouts can be a fun and motivating change of pace in your otherwise normal routine.

Stress and Sleep

Due to our current high-stress culture, we often remain in a state of chronic stress resulting in higher levels of cortisol a hormone that allows us to respond in fight or flight situations. However, a high and prolonged level of cortisol has a negative effect on blood pressure, blood sugar levels, and fat deposits.

Start with stress relieving exercises and activities, specifically deep breathing and meditation. Constructive strategies, like guided imagery and journaling, also reduce tension by processing experiences, clarifying thoughts and feelings, and developing self-knowledge.

Self-hypnosis or counseling can also help you learn to trigger your relaxation response, make healthy lifestyle changes, and overcome negative habits. And, fortunately, exercise, yoga and sex all serve a double function of burning calories and reducing stress.

These activities combine several obvious stress management factors: deep breathing, touch, emotional intimacy, endorphins and a physical workout. Overall, it elevates mood and lowers stress burning calories and activating the body's natural feel-good hormones.

You can also help your body balance its hunger and stress hormones by calming down and getting adequate, restful sleep. A Brigham Young University study found that women who sleep and wake at the same time every day have lower levels of body fat (Levine).

Cortisol levels naturally dip at bed time and increase over the night thus naturally waking you up in the morning. Chaotic sleep habits or even eating when you would normally be sleeping will upset your body's natural circadian rhythm, to which your body responds by secreting fat-storing hormones like cortisol. It is also important to get restful, uninterrupted sleep.

The fat-regulating hormone leptin is only produced during certain stages of sleep. Unsound sleep will disrupt leptin levels produced by fat cells. Inconsistent leptin levels mean that the body can't effectively keep track of its potential energy stored in its fat cells. To be on the safe side, your body will store calories rather than burn them.

There is still no agreement on the best or even a possible way to keep weight off long-term for the majority of people. But, everyone agrees that regular exercise and healthy eating habits improves health. The research of Steven Blair, professor of exercise science, epidemiology and biostatistics, indicates that "obese individuals who are fit have a death rate one half that of normal-weight people who are not fit" (Katz).

Dieting doesn't always lead to permanent weight loss, but neither does giving up dieting. For some ex-dieters, intuitive-eating does result in slimming down, but others just end up where they started. When you do reach your target weight, embrace your new body, address emotional issues in positive ways, and find appropriate strategies and sources of support.

Letting go of limiting beliefs is why the principles of Health at Every Size works. A moderate approach is more sustainable in the long run because it can become your lifestyle. Extreme no carbohydrate diets lead to muscle mass loss and no fat diets slow your metabolism. It isn't willpower or drive but patience that will help you obey the rules of fat loss.

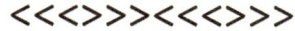

The Irresistible Combination of Sugar and Fat

So, you just love ice cream too much to give it up? You can't work without drinking a Coke? It would seem that fat-free ice cream and diet soda should solve all your fat problems, but you can't lose fat by just eliminating fat and reducing calories.

It isn't the fat in those cookies and donuts that is packing on the pounds. Sugar, in particular high fructose corn syrup, has a significant effect on insulin levels, fat storage and hunger. And, we crave more of it. Sweetened drinks as well as fatty and sugary foods, in particular fat and sugar in combination, affect your brain in a completely different way than natural food making it so much hard to resist overeating.

By itself, sugar offers no nutritional benefits. Since mammals, including humans, evolved in sugar-poor environments our sweet receptors are overly stimulated by our current sugar-rich diets, and the "happy feeling" we get from sugar in our reward centers of our brain overpower the self-control mechanisms that tell our bodies that we have had enough.

According to a report from the 2005–10 National Health and Nutrition Examination Survey database, Americans eat about 20 teaspoons of sugar a day getting more than 10% of their daily calories from added sugars—for men: 335 calories, women: 230 calories, boys: 362 calories, and girls: 282 calories (American Heart Association).

Of course, there is naturally occurring sugar in fruits, vegetables and milk, but added sugars affect insulin production and cause our fat cells to go into storage mode. It also prevents fat-burning since exercise burns the extra sugar first and then fat.

Your blood sugar tells your body whether to burn fat or store it

Your blood sugar level affects how energetic or hungry you feel. It also tells your body whether to burn fat or store it. When you eat complex carbohydrates, like starchy vegetables, breads and grains, your body processes the sugar slowly gradually increasing blood sugar levels during digestion.

In contrast, simple carbohydrates, or sugar and processed foods, are broken down quickly causing a steep increase in blood sugar. When your blood sugar level increases, your pancreas produces insulin to help regulate the sugar in your blood. Insulin transports sugar from your blood to your cells to be converted into energy.

It helps store glucose in the liver and muscles as glycogen and in fat cells as triglycerides. Higher levels of insulin tell your body that you have plenty of energy and to store fat instead of burning it. Since insulin is the fat storage hormone, it's actually impossible to burn body fat with this surge of insulin.

You'll be burning excess sugar, not fat. If blood sugar levels become very high and very suddenly, the body will release so much insulin that ultimately blood sugar drops below normal levels causing a sugar crash. Low levels of blood sugar cause you to feel tired and hungry, and our bodies respond by craving more sugar. Over time, the body becomes less sensitive to insulin, producing extra insulin, and using sugar more often for fat storage instead of energy.

When you skip a meal or diet, actually if you go more than 4-5 hours without eating, your blood sugar becomes unstable. So, when you do eat, your insulin levels will spike and, regardless of what you eat, store fat. The best ways to keep your blood sugar levels even are: eat breakfast, never skip a meal, and choose healthy snacks between meals that are high in fiber.

Avoid simple carbohydrates, processed foods and beverages with added sugar, as well as fat-free products that compensate for flavor with sugar. Without fat, sugar is absorbed into the blood even faster (Bass). Protein and fiber also slow sugar absorption and your rate of digestion.

This is why eating your fruit, which is high in fiber, is better than drinking fruit juice, which has strained out all the fiber. Omega 3 fatty acids, in wild fish, flax or chia seed and nuts, will also help maintain stable insulin levels. This is the most effective way to keep your metabolism high, prevent hunger pangs and binges.

Try to incorporate foods with a glycemic index below 55 like fruits and vegetables, including sweet potatoes but not russet potatoes, rice, oat bran bread and oatmeal (McCord). Overall, a low-glycemic diet prevents diabetes, headaches, heart disease, depression, yeast infection and cancer (Cox).

Some sugar is worse for you than other kinds of sugar

Glucose, or sugar, is a byproduct of photosynthesis and found naturally in fruits and vegetables. Our bodies can also produce glucose when needed. Naturally occurring sugars are found in milk, fruit and vegetables: lactose, fructose and glucose.

From the sunflower, we get another naturally occurring sweetener, Stevia, 300 times sweeter than sugar, which similarly affects blood sugar levels. Honey, however, has a different effect than sugar. Overall, honey helps improve blood lipids, lowers inflammatory markers and has little effect on blood sugar levels. However, since bees can only make so much honey, we get most of our sugar from sugar cane and sugar beets.

There are also a few artificial sweeteners that we have made. Most diet sodas and NutraSweet contain aspartame, a laboratory-created sugar alternative. Sucralose is another artificial sweetener, 600x sweeter than sugar. It is used in protein powers and Splenda. Saccharin was created back in the late 1890s but taken off the market when a study, which has not been replicated, linked it to an increased risk of cancer. So, while sugar in an apple is one thing, the extra sugar in your pasta or corn chips is another kind of problem.

Sucrose comes from the stems of sugar cane and sugar beet roots, which we process and refine into molasses and sugar. Refined sugars and syrups are then added to foods or beverages during processing or preparation as well.

It can be difficult to identify added sugars in foods. Current nutrition labels combine both added and naturally occurring sugars in the nutrition information, and the ingredient list can list each individual sugar to downplay its proportionally large presence.

Fruit juice concentrate and agave syrup sound less suspicious than high-fructose corn syrup and sucrose. But, in the end, it's all added sugar: Agave nectar, Brown sugar, Cane crystals, Cane sugar, Corn sweetener, Corn syrup, Crystalline fructose, Dextrose, Evaporated cane juice, Organic evaporated cane juice, Fructose, Fruit juice concentrates, Glucose, High-fructose corn syrup, Honey, Invert sugar, Lactose, Maltose, Malt syrup, Molasses, Raw sugar, Sucrose, Sugar, and Syrup.

The most commonly added sugars are regular table sugar and high fructose corn syrup. You should look for these and other common renaming of sugar on food labels. Any refinement process increases the effect the sugar or food has on blood sugar levels.

For example, agave nectar or agave syrup is sugar derived from the cactus plant, but it is made in the same way as high fructose corn syrup. It's highly processed and refined. While HFCS (high fructose corn syrup) is molecularly similar to regular sugar, consumption of food with this highly refined sugar results in greater weight gain than regular table sugar.

A Princeton University study found that rats gained significantly more weight consuming the same out of calories from HFCS as with table sugar. It also led to a larger increase in belly fat and circulating triglycerides (Kamb).

Besides sugar content, processed foods like white bread, French fries and other foods with a high glycemic index have the same effect on blood sugar level as glucose. While fruit combines sugar in its natural state with vitamins, minerals and fiber, it causes less of a blood sugar spike than table sugar, high fructose corn syrup or even potatoes.

Don't drink your sugar either

Candy and cookies shouldn't have to take all the blame. Soft drinks, sports drinks and fruit drinks contribute in large part to the added sugars in today's diet. With just one 12-ounce can of regular soda, you drink 8 teaspoons of added sugar and 130 calories. Drinking too many calories actually leads to weight gain more so than eating too many calories. Liquid calories are less satisfying, so people tend to consume more fluid calories.

For the most part, these kinds of drinks are sweetened with have high-fructose corn syrup. Drinks that are "sugar free" or artificially sweetened aren't necessarily healthy either. A study at the University of Texas Health Science Center found that people who drink diet sodas are at risk for weight gain, by as much as 41% (Fitday).

This is not because of excess calories. The heightened sweetness compared to its calorie-free content confuses the brain causing it to crave more calories (Loumarr). The carbonation might also bind to fat cells slowing down fat loss, and the extra air bloats the gastrointestinal tract slowing down digestion.

It has no nutritional value and depletes the body of nutrients necessary for strong bones and healthy weight loss, including vitamin A, calcium and magnesium. Between the sugar, caffeine, and carbonation, soft drinks contribute most obviously to tooth decay as well as weakened bones, obesity, and diabetes.

While the sugar and caffeine creates what can be a lifelong addiction to soda pop, if you give up even one soda a day, you would lose as much as 16 pounds of fat in one year. You can replace your soft drinks, sports drinks and fruit juices with water and tea. If you need a little bit of sweetness, add a slice of lemon, orange, lime or natural sweeteners like Stevia or honey.

The American Heart Association makes this recommendation for healthy levels of sugar consumption: "Typically, foods high in added sugars do not have nutrients the body needs and only contain extra calories. To get the nutrients you need, eat a diet that is rich in fruits, vegetables, fiber-rich whole grains, lean meats, fish, poultry, and low-fat or fat-free dairy product. No more than half of your daily discretionary calorie allowance should come from added sugars.

For most American women, this is no more than 100 calories per day (about 6 teaspoons). For men, it's no more than 150 calories per day (about 9 teaspoons). The American Heart Association recommends that all Americans consume no more than 450 calories (36 ounces) per week from sugar-sweetened beverages (based on a 2,000 calorie per day diet)" (American Heart Association).

Be on the lookout for foods with high fructose corn syrup, a high glycemic index and sweetened beverages, even diet sodas, which manipulate insulin production, signal fat storage and leave your tired and craving ever more sugar.

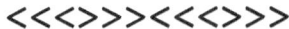

Extra bonus section tips

The fat loss benefits of adding organic foods to your diet

While the USDA makes no claims that organic foods are "safer, healthier, or more nutritious than conventional foods," it is clear that eating organic foods reduces exposure to pesticides, hormones and antibiotics.

Processed foods include food additives and food derivatives that affect insulin production, body inflammation and hunger cravings which all contribute to fat retention. They also are high in refined sugars and flour which are readily converted into glucose and fat.

Organic foods cannot be treated with any synthetic pesticide, sewage sludge, bioengineering or ionizing radiation (Zelman). While not always necessarily organic, a diet of whole grains, lean meats, fruits and vegetables and monounsaturated fats will contribute to fat loss. Complex carbohydrates, resistant starch, protein, antioxidants, and monounsaturated fats all play a role in fat loss by keeping your metabolism active, building fat burning muscle, and reducing inflammation.

Some fat is good for you

Not all fats are doomed to fill out your midsection. While there is a strong correlation between increased visceral fat and consuming saturated fats in meat and dairy, monounsaturated and polyunsaturated fats have an anti-inflammatory effect on the body. They also go towards building muscle mass.

The Institute of Medicine recommends that 20-35% of your daily calories come from fat, particularly monounsaturated and polyunsaturated fats (Renee). They promote healthy cholesterol levels, absorb fat-soluble vitamins, and provide essential fats necessary for healthy vision, neurological function and cardiovascular health.

Studies have found a correlation between a MUFA-rich diet and weight loss compared to a low-fat diet and weight gain. For example, a little bit of dark chocolate will curb cravings for salt, sweets and other unhealthy fats. The monounsaturated fats in just 1-ounce of dark chocolate will reduce cravings, stimulate your metabolism, and burn fat.

There are many great sources of monounsaturated fats that are also fiber, protein or calcium rich. You can get your calories, protein and monounsaturated fats in just a handful of dry and roasted nuts, particularly almonds, cashews, pistachios, pine nuts, contain protein. Or, you can add some monounsaturated fat to a salad or yogurt with a sprinkle of flaxseed, sesame and poppy seeds, or pumpkin and sunflower seeds.

Doubling as grains, chia seeds and quinoa are seeds high in monounsaturated fat. A little peanut oil in your stir fry, olive oil on your grilled fish, or seed oil instead of ranch dressing drizzled on your salad will also add healthy fats to your diet and reduce your consumption of saturated oils. For protein as well as monounsaturated fats, enjoy some salmon, cheese, and fiber-rich avocados. Grass-fed goat cheese and feta contain the highest content of these healthy fats that help you feel full and burn fat. Milk also has this same fatty acid as well as fat-burning calcium and hunger satisfying protein.

A pear a day, keeps the fat away

If it grows on a tree, bush, stalk or vine, you should be eating it. Fruits and vegetables are important sources of necessary minerals and vitamins, antioxidants and soluble fiber that help in fat loss. For example, you can find folate, a B-vitamin, in leafy green salads which correlates to weight loss eight times higher than a diet low in folate (Klein). You can add leafy greens like spinach and broccoli to your salads, omelets, and whole grain pastas.

Fruits and vegetables are also nutrient dense meaning that despite their volume they are low in calories. Because they are high in water and fiber, they make you feel full longer. This explains why eating fruit at the beginning of a meal reduces calorie intake by 15 percent (Perrine). For the same amount of calories, you can eat three cups of fresh strawberries and a cup of grapes, or you can eat a handful of potato chips and drink a soda.

You'll be hungry sooner after downing that coke and bag of chips. An orange is only 60 calories, but it will fill you up with fiber and help you eat less throughout the day. Grapefruit is 90% water but not only does it fill you up it also lowers your insulin, a fat-storage hormone. And, in just one pear you can get 15% of your daily recommended amount of fiber.

Another fat reducing quality of organic fruits and vegetables is the anti-inflammatory properties of anti-oxidants. For only 80 calories, one serving of blueberries has up to 4 grams of fiber as well as antioxidants important in fat loss.

A study at the University of California at Los Angeles found that the typical normal-weight person consumed about two servings of fruit a day, while the average overweight person ate just one a day (Perrine). You also get antioxidants in your tea and wine.

Tea hydrates your body just as water does but the antioxidants, or specifically catechins, also help to burn belly fat. Resveratrol, the antioxidant found in grape skin and thus wine, stops fat storage and boosts your calorie burn for up to an hour and a half. Overall, the antioxidants, vitamins and minerals in fruits and vegetables reduce your risk of cancer, diabetes, cholesterol and heart disease.

Good carbohydrates are high in resistant starch

Unlike other carbohydrates and simple sugars, resistant starch is not easily digested or absorbed as glucose in the small intestines. Thus, similar to insoluble and soluble fiber, it boosts metabolism and burns fat. It is found in seeds, legumes, whole grains, potatoes, leafy greens.

You can actually found the most resistant starch from bananas! A slightly green, medium-size banana has 12.5 grams of resistant starch. Even a ripe banana has 5 grams and half a cup of cooked plantains has 3 grams.

Next, beans are high in protein, fiber and resistant starch. A serving (½ cup) of white beans fills you up with fiber and 4 grams of resistant starch. In one serving of lentils, again rich in protein, you get 3.4 grams of resistant starch. The same amount of garbanzo beans gets you protein, fiber, iron, healthy fats, and 2 grams of resistant starch. Kidney beans are not only protein-rich but in one serving they also have 5 grams of fiber and 2 grams of resistant starch.

Beans don't have the saturated fat found in most meats while providing just as much protein (1 cup of black beans contains 15 grams of protein). Other grains, like oats, rice and barley, are also high in fiber and resistant starch. High in fiber, ½ cup of oats contains 4.6 grams of resistant starch.

While not as high, ½ cup of pearl barley has 2 grams of resistant starch and ½ cup of brown rice contains 1.7 g of resistant starch. Compare this to white rice and other processed grains that are quickly processed by the body into glucose. Plus, these foods are heavy and filling while low in calories (Klein).

Whole wheat, brown rice, whole grain breads, cereals and waffles are higher in fiber, thus more filling and nutritious. The calories in pastries and bagels go down fast because they are high in sugar and refined flour.

Processed foods like white bread, chips and sugary drinks and desserts increase inflammation in the body adding to the accumulation of belly fat. They also increase blood glucose levels and reduce the body's sensitivity to insulin, also resulting in fat storage.

Increasing protein and fiber, however, reduces the desire to binge eat, satiates hunger and fights increasing insulin resistance. 25-30% of the calories in protein is used in digestion, while only 6-8% of calories is used when eating simple carbohydrates and sugars.

A 2011 study found that an increase of 10 grams of soluble fiber a day decreased visceral fat by 3.7% loss over five years (Levine). In general, chips and dips are empty calories. Switch to salsa, hummus and bean dip on carrot sticks or whole wheat pita chips for a more satisfying and fat reducing snack.

Excitotoxins end up in our processed foods as food additives and derivatives as well as on our fresh produce from chemicals sprays, dips and baths. While they make the food tasty, it also turns off our natural sense of satiety, so we keep eating until the bag is empty.

Food additives are often allergenic causing insulin to spike adding to pre-diabetes factors (Salerno). And, last, the chemicals that help keep our produce without blemish also increase food cravings, water retention and weight gain. Some produce is more susceptible to pesticide residue including: apples, bell peppers, celery, cherries, grapes, lettuce, nectarines, peaches, pears, potatoes, spinach, and strawberries. Conversely, these fruits and vegetables naturally have the lowest pesticide residues: avocadoes, bananas, broccoli, cabbage, kiwifruit, mangoes, papayas, pineapple, onions, sweet corn and sweet peas (Zelman).

While it is almost impossible to get organic meat, you can look for hormone-free, grass fed, and wild caught milk, eggs and meat. Organic isn't the only way to reduce chemicals and additives in your food. Also look for hormone-free dairy products, locally grown produce, and grass fed and wild caught meat.

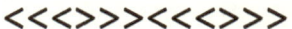

The connection between fat loss and sleep

Decrease Stress and Fat with Sleep

Early to bed and early to rise, makes a man healthy, wealthy and wise, or does it? When Benjamin Franklin popularized this proverb, he probably intended that a regular schedule contributes to a positive work ethic that affects your learning and earning potential as well as overall health. However, this has often been taken as an imperative only to work hard—off to work early.

In pursuit of the "wealthy" part of the proverb, we often work late too burning the midnight oil. As it turns out, though, not getting enough sleep is not wise at all. Restful sleep is important for recovering from daily physical and mental activities, but it also maintains the body's energy balance.

The majority of sleep is spent on tissue growth and repair, memory consolidation, and hormone regulation. Hormones essential for growth and development are also released. Some of these hormones also regulate appetite and fat retention, including the hunger hormones leptin and ghrelin as well as the stress hormone cortisol.

Sleep also supports a continued healthy immune system. When we are sleep-deprived, we are more prone to sickness, we may feel the need to eat more, and we may be more stressed. All of these factors can contribute to weight gain and hinder fat loss.

Not sleeping enough makes you hungrier

It's not uncommon to not get enough sleep—30% of Americans sleep less than six hours a night. A longitudinal study that looked at almost 70,000 women over 16 years found that "short sleep duration is associated with a modest increase in future weight gain and incident obesity" (Patel).

Regardless of exercise and diet, women who slept six hours gained weight and women who slept five hours or less gained even more. These women were 30% more likely to gain belly fat than those who slept seven or more hours.

While sleeping too much is also a risk factor, the weight gain is more likely due to a less active lifestyle. One of the explanations for this correlation between short sleep duration and weight gain is related to how sleep regulates the hunger hormones, leptin and ghrelin.

We know that a diet high in complex carbohydrates or protein suppresses ghrelin, one of the body's hormones that induce hunger, more effectively than a diet high in fat. The stomach releases ghrelin signaling hunger to the brain. Ghrelin levels are higher in children with anorexia nervosa and lower in children who are obese.

However, levels of ghrelin have also been found to be higher among sleep deprived children (Magee). Sleep has a significant effect on leptin and ghrelin levels in people who sleep only four hours a night. After just two days of sleep deprivation, they experienced an 18% drop in leptin and 28% rise in ghrelin (Mercola).

A drop in leptin signals a need to conserve fat stores and an increase in ghrelin signals hunger in general. Since the brain is fueled by glucose, when sleep-deprived, it searches for carbohydrates. The sleep-deprived subjects chose to eat sweet and starchy foods over vegetables and dairy products. In essence, sleep deprivation puts your body into a pre-diabetic state as well as conserving fat and making you hungrier.

Stress enlarges your fat cells

Sleep deprivation affects not only leptin and ghrelin but also cortisol levels, the stress hormone. Cortisol plays a role in bone growth, blood pressure control, and immune system and nervous system function. It is thus named the stress hormone because it is secreted in higher levels during the body's fight or flight response to stress.

When under stress, the pituitary gland in the brain releases a hormone called adrenocorticotropic or ACTH. The adrenal gland responds by producing a steroid hormone (cortisol), which increases the body's ability to respond to the stressful situation.

A small increase of cortisol results in a quick burst of energy, increased immunity, lower pain sensitivity, heightened memory function and helps maintain homeostasis in the body (Wisse). This is all very important in life threatening situations but not as useful when dealing with the chronic stress of demanding work schedules, sleep deprivation and overstimulation.

Though not as obvious as holding onto fat or inducing hunger, cortisol plays an important part in fat loss or gain. Cortisol regulates blood pressure, inflammatory response, insulin release for blood sugar maintenance, and proper glucose metabolism. It also affects the metabolism of fats, carbohydrates and proteins.

High and prolonged levels of cortisol is associated with high blood pressure, decreased bone density and muscle tissue, impaired cognitive performance, suppressed thyroid function, and lowered immunity and inflammatory responses (Scott). It also results in increased abdominal fat and thus heart attacks, strokes and metabolic syndrome.

While stress eating accounts for some of the weight gain, even those who respond to stress by not eating also retain fat. That is because cortisol enlarges your fat cells and increases the amount of visceral fat in your body regardless of what you eat.

Reduce your stress

Due to our current high-stress environments and culture, we often remain in a state of chronic stress. This results in unhealthy cortisol levels. You must help prompt your body's relaxation response so that the body does not remain in a constant state of flight or fight.

Some people eat when they are stressed. This is because they secrete higher levels of cortisol in response to stress. They also tend to eat food higher in carbohydrates. If you are biologically more sensitive to stress, stress management and a low-stress lifestyle will play a larger factor in your weight loss.

Start with stress relieving exercising and activities like listening to music or gardening but also specifically deep breathing and meditation. Guided imagery, journaling, and self-hypnosis can help you manage stress.

These are all constructive strategies to process traumatic experiences, clarify thoughts and feelings, and gain self-knowledge. It can also help you fight tension. Self-hypnosis or counseling can help you learn to trigger your relaxation response, make healthy lifestyle changes like setting boundaries or decluttering, and overcome negative habits like smoking or binge eating. And, fortunately, exercise, yoga and sex all serve a double function of burning calories and reducing stress.

Due to the strength building poses and deep breathing of yoga, postmenopausal women who participated in regular yoga for 16 weeks reported a significant reduction in belly fat (Levine). Likewise, sex combines several obvious stress management factors:

deep breathing, touch, emotional intimacy, endorphins and a physical workout.

Overall, it elevates mood and lowers stress. Exercise also burns calories and activates the body's natural feel-good hormones. Whether you find some time to relax with friends, exercise to blow off steam, or utilize counseling, developing and maintaining a low-stress lifestyle will prevent unnecessary fat gain.

Get a good night's sleep

You can also help your body balance its hunger and stress hormones by calming down and getting adequate, restful sleep. An oft-cited Brigham Young University study found that women who sleep and wake at the same time every day have lower levels of body fat (Levine).

Cortisol levels naturally dip at bed time and increase over the night thus naturally waking you up in the morning. Chaotic sleep habits or even eating when you would normally be sleeping will upset your body's natural circadian rhythm, to which your body responds by secreting fat-storing hormones like cortisol. It is also important to get restful, uninterrupted sleep.

The fat-regulating hormone leptin is only produced during certain stages of sleep. Unsound sleep will disrupt leptin levels produced by fat cells. Inconsistent leptin levels mean that the body can't effectively keep track of its potential energy stored in its fat cells.

To be on the safe side, your body will store calories rather than burn them. So, you can set yourself up for the best possible sleep by improving your bedtime routines several hours after exercising, eating or consuming caffeine. Turn off your electronic devices, close the blinds, put on some white noise, and tuck yourself in for the night. When possible, don't set your alarm and let your body naturally reset its internal clock.

Regardless of how much you diet or exercise, not getting enough sleep will result in more belly fat. Sleep habits directly influence the accumulation of visceral fat and thus weight gain around your abdominal area.

Belly fat contributes to heart disease, cardiovascular disease, type 2 diabetes and other chronic diseases. Restful, regular sleep gives your body enough time to regulate hunger hormones like leptin and ghrelin which tell your body if you have enough energy reserves and if you need to eat more.

Not sleeping enough makes you hungrier. If your body does not have the proper amount of time to recover from daily stresses, your body will continue in a state of chronic stress with higher and more prolonged levels of cortisol which regulate glucose metabolism, insulin levels and fat storage. So, it's time to stop stressing out and get a good night's sleep. You'll find you're in a better mood, well-rested, and thinner.

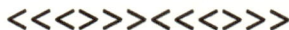

Cabbage based liquids for fat loss

Drink Fat Away with Cabbage

Cabbage has been around for more than a thousand years. It became a prominent part of European cuisine in the Middle Ages, including sauerkraut, coleslaw, stuffed cabbage, corned beef and cabbage, sandwiches, and soups.

It is a good source of vitamins A, B, C, E, K, folate and dietary fiber. In the 1980s, the cabbage soup diet gained some traction as a short-term weight-loss diet, inspiring many other crash diets. It is a low-fat, low-calorie seven day plan meant for quick weight loss.

In essence, you can eat as much cabbage soup as you want during the week and specific additional foods on other days. People report having lost up to 10 pounds of weight in one week, however because it is physiologically impossible to loss that much fat within one week most of the weight lost is water.

As an alternative to cutting your daily intake to near-starvation caloric intake and forcing down bowls of cabbage soup, incorporate cabbage juice into your daily diet. Cabbage does have fat burning qualities as well as vitamins, minerals and dietary fiber that will contribute to an overall healthy fat-burning diet.

The Original Cabbage Soup Diet

This week-long diet regiments seven days of all you can eat fat-free cabbage soup with additional food designated on certain days. At little more than 70 calories, besides cabbage, a bowl of cabbage soup can include: green onions, green peppers, tomatoes, carrots, mushrooms, celery, chicken stock and water.

On the fruit, vegetable and soup only days, this diet subsists on 500-800 calories. Only three days allow a more normal daily caloric intake of up to 1500 additional calories from meat, milk or potatoes. Unfortunately, most of the beneficial fiber is cooked out of the cabbage. The diet allows only for water, tea, unsweetened fruit juices, and a few additional food items (Tomovich).

Day 1: Cabbage soup and fruit (no bananas)

Day 2: Cabbage soup, leafy greens and a medium potato with butter

Day 3: Cabbage soup, fruits and vegetables (no potatoes or bananas)

Day 4: Cabbage soup, up to 8 bananas and unlimited skim milk

Day 5: Cabbage soup and 10-20 oz of beef or skinless chicken and up to 6 tomatoes

Day 6: Cabbage soup, vegetables (no potatoes) and beef (even steak)

Day 7: Cabbage soup, brown rice and vegetables

To make it tastier and less bland, you can add spices like coriander and mustard, garlic, thyme and marjoram, caraway seeds or bay leaf. If you add salt and pepper, you run the risk of consuming too much sodium. A piece of rye bread or smoked meat will add a lot of flavor to the soup, but it technically isn't allowed by the diet.

Since the cabbage soup diet is low-fat, high-fiber and so low in calories, of course you lose weight. It certainly is a quick fix to drop weight for a special event, and you only have to stick to it for one week. However, for the most part, you lose water weight and even lean tissue.

The drastically limited calories will adversely disrupt the normal balance of hormones regulating insulin, fat retention and hunger. It is also low in complex carbohydrates, protein, vitamins and minerals, so you should not consume a cabbage soup diet for more than a week.

Cabbage, especially cooked cabbage, is not completely absorbed in the intestines ending up in the colon where bacteria break it down creating gas. So, be prepared for some cabbage-induced farts. In general, a low calorie diet can cause lightheadedness, headaches, dizziness, and general lack of energy for daily activities and exercise.

Lovisa Nilsson, a nutritionist quoted in magazine Marie Claire, said: "Cabbage soup is nutritionally unbalanced as a meal, and it is vital we consume essential nutrients such as proteins, vitamins B and even healthy fats.

By following this diet for a lengthy period of time, you are depriving your body of the nutrients it needs and thus defeating any long-term health benefits....Supplement the soup with rye bread and some form of protein" (Ramsdale). Very popular in Austria and Russia, cabbage soup often also includes beans and smoked meat.

The Health and Fat Loss Benefits of Cabbage

Just because the week-long cabbage diet has some serious health disadvantages, does not meant that cabbage itself is not good for fat loss. There are three major varieties of cabbage—the green, red-purple, and Savoy (yellowish green). The red-to-purple pigmentation in cabbage results in more nutrients.

For a vegetable, it contains impressive amounts of calcium, iron, iodine, potassium, sulfur, and phosphorus. In general, cabbage is rich in anti-oxidants, including vitamins A, B1, B2, B6, C, E, K and folate thus it is highly promoted as a cancer-fighting super food.

It is also a rich source of phytonutrients fighting harmful toxins and hormones, producing more antibodies, and boosting immune defenses (Ding). And, like other vegetables, it is high in dietary fiber and low in calories.

Fresh cabbage has demonstrated its usefulness as a supplement in treating cancer and ulceration in the digestive tracts. It contains a compound known as histidine that regulates T-cells in the immune system, and thus is useful in treating allergies. Sulforaphine also protects cells against carcinogens.

The chlorophyll in cabbage is good for blood building and thus useful in relation to anemia. It can also be used to treat sores on the outside and inside. Topical use of cabbage leaves on enlarged and swollen breasts, particularly due to nursing, is a soothing and natural alternative to other medicines. Likewise, cabbage leaves can be used to treat skin wounds, blisters, sores, burns, ulcers and psoriasis.

Cabbage also stimulates bowel movements, and the amino acid glutamine gently cleanses the digestive system. The high sulfur, chlorine and iodine content effectively cleanse the mucus membranes of the stomach and intestinal tracts as well as repairing ulcers, detoxifying and regenerating the digestive system in general.

Cabbage contributes to fat loss through the same vitamins, minerals and fiber that other vegetables have. Substances in cabbage help prevent the conversion of sugar and carbohydrates into fat. Specifically, the vitamin B complex in cabbage is known for acting as a catalyst for high metabolism of energy.

You can also add a little bit of vinegar or lemon juice to your cabbage to burn fat. A 2009 Japanese study found that significant visceral fat loss resulted after eight weeks of consuming 1-2 tablespoons of vinegar daily (Levine). Lemon juice and other acidic foods increase carbohydrate combustion by 20-40% (Men's Fitness). The acid tempers insulin spikes, slows the digestion process, and produces proteins that burn fat. This is why fermented foods like pickles, yogurt and kim chee are also good options.

Substitute High Calorie Drinks with Cabbage Juice

To lose weight and fat, substitute high calorie drinks and fruit juices with cabbage juice. Depending on whether you use green or red cabbage, a 1-cup serving of cabbage juice is 22-28 calories with 0.09-0.14 grams of fat. Drinking just one glass of cabbage juice a week over the year can lead to 1.5 pounds of fat loss. Cabbage juice has 1.9-2.2 grams of dietary fiber which is 5-9% of the recommended daily fiber intake (Dannie). However, you need to add back the fiber after the juicing process.

To make one cup of cabbage juice, you need 1 cup of chopped cabbage and ¼ cup water. You can store cabbage juice for up to five days in the refrigerator. One cup of cabbage juice is one-third to one-half of your recommended vegetable intake. In general, the smaller varieties of cabbage taste better.

Purple cabbage is also sweeter than the green or Savoy varieties. But, for taste, you can always temper the strong taste of cabbage by juicing it with apple, beet, carrot, celery, cucumber, lemon (and lemon peel), and spinach. For digestion, cabbage sprouts are easier to digest and higher in nutrients. Since cooked cabbage is harder to digest than raw or juiced, cabbage juice is more beneficial than cabbage soup. As soon as it is cut, halved or shredded, cabbage begins to lose its nutrients. So, to prevent loss of vitamins, refrigerate your cabbage in a perforated plastic bag. Start small and slowly increase how much cabbage juice you drink overall.

Like grapefruit and celery, cabbage doesn't necessarily burn fat. No food burns fat, however the vitamins, minerals and fiber contribute to healthy digestion, metabolism, and inflammatory and immune responses that affect fat loss or retention.

While the cabbage soup diet might be one way to jump start your weight loss plans, incorporating cabbage overall into an already healthy diet will benefit your weight loss efforts. In your daily meals, you can include some balanced meals of cabbage soup with meat and rye bread as well as drinking more cabbage juices throughout the day.

Combined with a healthy eating and exercise plan, cabbage based liquids will help you lose weight, not water or muscle mass, and keep it off.

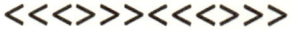

References

Body Fat. (2012). *Segen's Medical Dictionary*. Retrieved from http://medical-dictionary.thefreedictionary.com/

Body Fat (2012). *Medical Dictionary for the Health Professions and Nursing*. Retrieved from http://medical-dictionary.thefreedictionary.com/

Fat. (2007). *Dorland's Medical Dictionary for Health Consumers*. Retrieved from http://medical-dictionary.thefreedictionary.com/

Metabolism. (2009). *Mosby's Medical Dictionary*. 8th ed. Retrieved from http://medical-dictionary.thefreedictionary.com/

Bouchard, Claude, Ph.D., and Angelo Tremblay, Ph.D. (1990). The Response to Long-Term Overfeeding in Identical Twins. *The New England Journal of Medicine*, 322, 1477-1482. http://www.nejm.org/doi/full/10.1056/NEJM199005243222101

Parker-Pope, Tara. (2011, Dec 31). The Fat Trap. *The New York Times*. Retrieved from http://www.nytimes.com/2012/01/01/magazine/tara-parker-pope-fat-trap.html?pagewanted=all&_r=0

Proietto, Joseph, Ph.D. (2011). Long-Term Persistence of Hormonal Adaptations to Weight Loss. *The New England Journal of Medicine*, 365, 1597-1604. http://www.nejm.org/doi/full/10.1056/NEJMoa1105816

U.S. Dept. of Health and Human Services, U.S. Dept. of Agriculture. (2010). *Dietary Guidelines for Americans, 2010*. Washington, D.C. Retrieved from http://www.health.gov/dietaryguidelines/dga2010/dietaryguidelines2010.pdf

Collins, Sonya. The Truth about Belly Fat. WebMD Feature. Retrieved from http://www.webmd.com/diet/features/the-truth-about-belly-fat/

Doheny, Kathleen. The Truth about Fat. WebMD Feature. Retrieved from http://www.webmd.com/diet/features/the-truth-about-fat

Harvard Health. (2006). Abdominal Fat and What to Do about It. http://www.health.harvard.edu/newsweek/Abdominal-fat-and-what-to-do-about-it.htm

Klein, Samuel, M.D. (2004). Absence of an Effect of Liposuction on Insulin Action and Risk Factors for Coronary Heart Disease. *The New England Journal of Medicine,* 350, 2549-2557. http://www.nejm.org/doi/full/10.1056/NEJMoa033179

Magee, Elaine, R.D. Your 'Hunger Hormones.' Web MD Weight Loss Clinic Feature. Retrieved from http://www.webmd.com/diet/features/your-hunger-hormones

Rossi, Carey. (2014). 11 Reasons Why You're Not Losing Belly Fat. Retrieved from http://www.foxnews.com/health/2014/05/10/11-reasons-why-youre-not-losing-belly-fat/

Johnson, Chalene. (2012, May 25). 10 Eating Habits of the Highly Successful and Fit. *Push.* Wavebreak Media/Thinkstock. Retrieved from http://www.womenshealthmag.com/weight-loss/healthy-eating-habits

Men's Fitness. (2014). 101 Ways to Burn Belly Fat Fast. Retrieved from http://www.mensfitness.com/weight-loss/burn-fat-fast/101-ways-lose-your-gut

National Weight Control Registry. NWCR Facts. http://www.nwcr.ws/research/)

Harvard Health. (2006, Dec). Abdominal Fat and What to Do about It. http://www.health.harvard.edu/newsweek/Abdominal-fat-and-what-to-do-about-it.htm

Health.com (2014) 24 Fat-Burning Ab Exercises (No Crunches!) Retrieved from http://www.health.com/health/gallery/0,,20664616_6,00.html

Mayo Clinic. (2013, June 8) Belly fat in women: Taking — and keeping — it off. Retrieved from http://www.mayoclinic.org/healthy-living/womens-health/in-depth/belly-fat/art-20045809

Men's Fitness. (2014). 101 Ways to Burn Belly Fat Fast. Retrieved from http://www.mensfitness.com/weight-loss/burn-fat-fast/101-ways-lose-your-gut

Klein, Sarah. (2013, Jan 9). Best Superfoods for Weight Loss. http://www.myenergynutrition.com/blog/best-superfoods-for-weight-loss

Levine, Hallie. (2014). 9 Proven Ways to Lose Stubborn Belly Fat. http://www.prevention.com/weight-loss/weight-loss-tips/new-research-how-lose-belly-fat

Perrine, Stephen & Leah Flickinger. (2014, Feb 5). Eat More, Lose More Weight. Women's Health Magazine. http://www.womenshealthmag.com/weight-loss/eat-and-lose-weight

Renee, Janet. (2014, Feb 7). MUFA List of Foods. http://www.livestrong.com/article/298213-mufa-list-of-foods/

Salerno, John, Linda Eckhardt & James Beard. (2010, March 18). Why I Recommend Organic Foods to my Weight Loss Patients. Huffington Post. http://www.huffingtonpost.com/dr-john-salerno/why-i-recommend-organic-f_b_403348.html

Zelman, Kathleen. (2007, Aug 10). Organic Food—Is 'Natural' Worth the Extra Cost? Web MD. http://www.webmd.com/food-recipes/features/organic-food-is-natural-worth-the-extra-cost

Levine, Hallie. (2014). 9 Proven Ways to Lose Stubborn Belly Fat. http://www.prevention.com/weight-loss/weight-loss-tips/new-research-how-lose-belly-fat

Magee, Elaine. Your 'Hunger Hormones.' WebMD. http://www.webmd.com/diet/features/your-hunger-hormones

Mercola, Joseph. (2010, Mar 16). How Much do you Need to Sleep Every Night to Prevent Weight Gain? http://articles.mercola.com/sites/articles/archives/2010/03/16/poor-sleep-habits-lead-to-fat-gain.aspx

Patel, Sanjay. (2006, Apr 12). Association between Reduced Sleep and Weight Gain in Women. American Journal of Epidemiology. http://aje.oxfordjournals.org/content/164/10/947.full

Scott, Elizabeth. (2014, Dec 18). Cortisol and Stress: How to Stay Healthy. http://www.stress.about.com/od/stresshealth/a/cortisol.htm

Wisse, Brent. (2013, Nov 7). Cortisol Blood Test. United States National Library of Medicine. Medline Plus. http://www.nlm.nih.gov/medlineplus/ency/article/003693.htm

Dannie, Marie. (2014, Jul 25). How to Drink Cabbage Juice for Weight Loss. Livestrong. http://www.livestrong.com/article/420167-how-to-drink-cabbage-juice-for-weight-loss

Ding, Sarah. (2005-2014). Health Benefits of Cabbage. Retrieved from http://juicing-for-health.com/basic-nutrition/healing-vegetables/healt-benefits-of-cabbage.html

Levine, Hallie. (2014). 9 Proven Ways to Lose Stubborn Belly Fat. http://www.prevention.com/weight-loss/weight-loss-tips/new-research-how-lose-belly-fat

Men's Fitness. (2014). 101 Ways to Burn Belly Fat Fast. Retrieved from http://www.mensfitness.com/weight-loss/burn-fat-fast/101-ways-lose-your-gut

Ramsdale, Suzannah. (2014, Nov 25). Cabbage Soup Diet: Everything You Need to Know. Marie Claire. http://www.marieclaire.co.uk/blogs/433629/cabbage-soup-diet.html

Tomovich, Maryann. (2013, Dec 9). The Cabbage Soup Diet. Web MD. http://www.webmd.com/diet/cabbage-soup-diet

Johnson, Chalene. (2012, May 25). 10 Eating Habits of the Highly Successful and Fit. *Push*. Wavebreak Media/Thinkstock. Retrieved from http://www.womenshealthmag.com/weight-loss/healthy-eating-habits

Men's Fitness. (2014). 101 Ways to Burn Belly Fat Fast. Retrieved from http://www.mensfitness.com/weight-loss/burn-fat-fast/101-ways-lose-your-gut

Women's Health. (2013). 10 Health Snacks for Weight Loss. Retrieved from http://www.womenshealthmag.com/weight-loss/healthy-snacking

Zelman, Kathleen. (2008, March 7). How to Lose Weight while Eating More Food. WebMD Weight Loss Clinic. Retrieved from http://www.webmd.com/diet/features/how-to-lose-eight-while-eating-more-food

Bass, Thomas. (2015). How Blood Sugar Levels Affect Weight Loss. http://www.gulfcoastbariatrics.com/obesity-and-health/how-blood-sugar-levels-affect-weight-loss

Collins, Sonya. The Truth about Belly Fat. WebMD Feature. Retrieved from http://www.webmd.com/diet/features/the-truth-about-belly-fat/

Marteski, Steve. (2015). 5 Easy Ways to Lose Body Fat http://www.active.com/fitness/articles/5-easy-ways-to-lose-body-fat

Mirlenbrink, Karen. (2015). Melt Away Fat with Interval Training http://www.active.com/fitness/articles/melt-away-fat-with-interval-training

Women's Health. (2015). How Does Your Body Burn Fat? http://www.active.com/fitness/articles/how-does-your-body-burn-fat

Carneiro, Alex. (2014, Jan 7) 8 Fat Loss Blunders http://www.bodybuilding.com/fun/fat-loss-blunders-8-reasons-youre-not-losing-body-fat.html

Dhillon, Kisar. (2015). Understand Your BMI and Body Fat Percentage.   Active.com.

http://www.active.com/fitness/articles/understand-your-bmi-and-body-fat-percentage

Kelly, Diana. (2015). Diet and Fitness Rumors that Slow Weight Loss http://www.prevention.com/weight-loss/weight-loss-tips/10-diet-and-fitness-rumors-slow-weight-loss

Mercola, Joseph. (2010, Mar 16). How Much do you Need to Sleep Every Night to Prevent Weight Gain? http://articles.mercola.com/sites/articles/archives/2010/03/16/poor-sleep-habits-lead-to-fat-gain.aspx

Patel, Sanjay. (2006, Apr 12). Association between Reduced Sleep and Weight Gain in Women. American Journal of Epidemiology. http://aje.oxfordjournals.org/content/164/10/947.full

Wisse, Brent. (2013, Nov 7). Cortisol Blood Test. United States National Library of Medicine. Medline Plus. http://www.nlm.nih.gov/medlineplus/ency/article/003693.htm

Harding, Kate. (2007-2010). Illustrated BMI Categories. Flickr Photoset. https://www.flickr.com/photos/77367764@N00/sets/72157602199008819/.

Katz, Mandy. (2009, Jul 15). Tossing Out the Diet and Embracing the Fat. The New York Times. http://www.nytimes.com/2009/07/16/health/nutrition/16skin.html?_r=0

Macrae, Fiona. (2011, Oct 21). Being Too Skinny Damages Fertility More than Obesity. Daily Mail. http://www.dailymail.co.uk/health/article-2051512/Being-skinny-damages-fertility-obesity.html

Pearson, Judith. (2014). Cope with the Mental Challenges of Weight Loss and Embrace your New Body. http://expertbeacon.com/cope-mental-challenges-weight-loss-and-embrace-your-new-body/#.VIyUjTHF-So

Sifferlin, Alexandra. (2014, Mar 10). The Hidden Dangers of 'Skinny Fat." Time. http://time.com/14407/the-hidden-dangers-of-skinny-fat/?xid=rodale

Johnson, Chalene. (2012, May 25). 10 Eating Habits of the Highly Successful and Fit. *Push*. Wavebreak Media/Thinkstock. Retrieved from http://www.womenshealthmag.com/weight-loss/healthy-eating-habits

Kamb, Steve. (2013, Jun 17). Why Sugar is Worse than Darth Vadar.   Nerd   Fitness. http://www.nerdfitness.com/blog/2013/06/17/everything-you-need-to-know-about-sugar/

Katz, Mandy. (2009, Jul 15). Tossing Out the Diet and Embracing the Fat. The New York Times. http://www.nytimes.com/2009/07/16/health/nutrition/16skin.html?_r=0

Levine, Hallie. (2014). 9 Proven Ways to Lose Stubborn Belly Fat.   http://www.prevention.com/weight-loss/weight-loss-tips/new-research-how-lose-belly-fat

Mirlenbrink, Karen. (2015). Melt Away Fat with Interval Training   http://www.active.com/fitness/articles/melt-away-fat-with-interval-training

Rossi, Carey. (2014). 11 Reasons Why You're Not Losing Belly Fat.   Retrieved   from http://www.foxnews.com/health/2014/05/10/11-reasons-why-youre-not-losing-belly-fat/

Salerno, John, Linda Eckhardt & James Beard. (2010, March 18). Why I Recommend Organic Foods to my Weight Loss Patients. Huffington Post. http://www.huffingtonpost.com/dr-john-salerno/why-i-recommend-organic-f_b_403348.html

Dryden-Edwards, Roxanne. (2014, Dec 11). Emotional Eating. http://www.medicinenet.com/emotional_eating/article.htm

May Clinic Staff. (2012, Dec 1). Weight Loss: Gain Control of Emotional   Eating   http://www.mayoclinic.org/healthy-living/weight-loss/in-depth/weight-loss/art-20047342

Goad, Kimberly. (2012, Apr 17). Emotional Eating: The Trick to Staying Slim. http://www.foxnews.com/health/2012/04/16/emotional-eating-trick-to-staying-slim/

Gupta, Sumati. (2012, Mar 23). Is your brain wired to make you crave food when you're sad? Retrieved from http://www.bingeeatingbulimia.com/blog/2012/3/23/is-your-brain-wired-to-make-you-crave-food-when-youre-sad.html

Manning, Joy. (2014, Jul 28). Emotional Eating: What Helps http://www.webmd.com/diet/features/emotional-eating

American Heart Association. (2014, May 19). Frequently Asked Questions about Sugar. http://www.heart.org/HEARTORG/GettingHealthy/NutritionCenter/HealthyDietGoals/Frequently-Asked-Questions-About-Sugar_UCM_306725_Article.jsp

Bass, Thomas. (2015). How Blood Sugar Levels Affect Weight Loss. http://www.gulfcoastbariatrics.com/obesity-and-health/how-blood-sugar-levels-affect-weight-loss

Cox, Carrie. (2013, Jan 28). How Does Blood Sugar Affect Weight-Loss? http://www.slcfitcollective.com/carries-blog/how-does-blood-sugar-affect-weight-loss

Fitday. (2013). Want to Lose Weight Fast? Cut out Soda from Your Diet. http://www.fitday.com/fitness/weight-loss/want-to-lose-weight-fast-cut-out-soda-from-your-diet.html

Loumarr, Ess. (2013, Oct 21). How Much Weight Can You Lose by Not Drinking Soda? http://www.livestrong.com/article/406821-how-much-weight-can-you-lose-by-not-drinking-soda/

McCord, Holly. (2011, Nov). Your Guide to the Glycemic Index. http://www.prevention.com/food/food-remedies/glycemic-index-and-blood-sugar-levels

www.ingramcontent.com/pod-product-compliance
Lightning Source LLC
Chambersburg PA
CBHW050357290526
45786CB00003B/1031